MEDICAL IDENTITIES

SOCIAL IDENTITIES

General Editors: Shirley Ardener, Tamara Dragadze and Jonathan Webber

Based on a prominent Oxford University seminar founded over two decades ago by the social anthropologist Edwin Ardener, this series focuses on the ethnic, historical, religious, and other elements of culture that give rise to a social sense of belonging, enabling individuals and groups to find meaning both in their own social identities and in what differentiates them from others. Each volume is based on one specific theme that brings together contemporary material from a variety of cultures.

MEDICAL IDENTITIES

HEALTH, WELL-BEING AND PERSONHOOD

Edited by
Kent Maynard

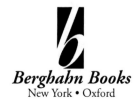

Berghahn Books
New York • Oxford

First published in 2007 by
Berghahn Books
www.berghahnbooks.com

©2007 Kent Maynard

Library of Congress Cataloging-in-Publication Data

Medical identities : health, well-being and personhood / edited by Kent Maynard.
     p. ; cm. -- (Social identities ; v. 2)
Includes bibliographical references and index.
ISBN-13: 978-1-84545-038-0 (hbk.) -- ISBN-13: 978-1-84545-100-4 (pbk.)
1. Physicians--Cross-cultural studies. 2. Medicine--Cross-cultural studies. 3. Professional socialization. 4. Group identity. 5. Self. I. Maynard, Kent, 1947- II. Series.
[DNLM: 1. Health Personnel--psychology. 2. Cross-Cultural Comparison. 3. Ethnic Groups--psychology. 4. Self Concept. 5. Social Identification. W 87 M489 2007]

R727.M48 2007
616--dc22

2007007397

British Library Cataloguing in Publication Data

A catalogue record for this book is available from the British Library

Printed in the United States on acid-free paper

ISBN-10: 1-84545-038-8   ISBN-13: 978-1-84545-038-0   (hardback)
ISBN-10: 1-84545-100-7   ISBN-13: 978-1-84545-100-4   (paperback)

Contents

LIST OF ILLUSTRATIONS

ACKNOWLEDGEMENTS

The essays in this volume grew out of a 'Seminar on Medical Identity' during Hilary Term 2003 at the Institute of Social and Cultural Anthropology, University of Oxford. I am grateful to the co-conveners of the Seminar, Shirley Ardener, Ian Fowler and Elisabeth Hsu, for their initiative and leadership in organising the Seminar. I am especially indebted to Shirley Ardener, as the General Editor of the series Social Identity, published with Berghahn Books, who invited me to edit this volume, the second in the series. Finally, let me thank our reader, Dr. Tamara Dragsolze, for her generous commentary and suggestions for each of the chapters.

INTRODUCTION

WORKING AT THERAPEUTIC PERSONHOOD

Kent Maynard

> As individuals express their life, so they are.
>
> Marx and Engels 1970: 42.

> [T]he cultural formative activity which is entailed in … work
> and identity unfolds in a social arena which positions [workers] … in
> fields of power and which should be seen as both historically
> and socially mediated.
>
> Ulin 2002: 694.

This is a book about 'medical identity'. Illness, and misfortune generally, are ubiquitous. It is no accident, then, that healing and other forms of giving or taking care are equally universal. Ironically, however, relatively little attention has been paid to the identity of those who heal or promote well-being. A significant, though partial, exception comes in regard to spirit possession, where there is a growing literature on mediums and personhood (and/or the body), at times in relation to wider issues of individual and social health or welfare. Much, though certainly not all, of the work on spirit possession and personhood, or larger issues of identity, comes from sub-Saharan Africa (e.g., Boddy 1989; Comaroff 1994: 306f.; Corin 1998; Lan 1985; Masquelier 2001; Rasmussen 1995). Yet, with the exception of these and other departures (e.g., Shaw 2002), a good deal of scholarship may either overlook 'medical identity' or implicitly assume that it is relatively unproblematic.

Of course, medical practice comes in many guises: healing may be highly professional and specialised, or far less formal; some societies are most concerned with prevention, while others focus on intervention. Based on rich and wide-ranging ethnographic data, the essays in this collection consider both the self-fashioning and collective work of identity formation involved in healing and the pursuit of well-being. Whether as acupuncturists, physicians, diviners or mid-wives, among many others, care giving, in Ulin's terms (2002: 694), is socially mediated. All the authors ask, as well, about how lay people view medical identities, and how these identities are influenced by wider social and cultural factors. As the essays demonstrate, class, gender, sexuality, ethnicity, or state policy may all have a formative and/or formidable influence shaping cultural definitions of health and well-being, how they are delivered, and the character and prestige of those who contribute to our welfare in society.

Locating identity

In thinking about 'medical identity' let me begin with the noun, returning later to the adjective 'medical'. Identity is one of those concepts that simultaneously face in two directions – towards the individual and towards the group – at once opening on to an exterior world of sociality (and even the cosmos), yet equally personal. Even modified by the adjective 'social', the term 'social identity' implies both membership in a group and something about the individual as a self and as a person. It may be a truism to say that human beings are social; yet, under-standing the myriad ways in which we 'embody' larger groups, while at the same time helping constitute them, remains deeply fascinating.

For Karl Marx and Fredrich Engels, that process is inextricably tied to work: not to oversimplify, we are what we do. Or, as they write in *The German Ideology*,

> As individuals express their life, so they are. What they are, therefore, coincides with their production, both with *what* they produce and with *how* they produce. The nature of individuals thus depends on the material conditions determining their production. (1970: 42; emphasis original)

Our very awareness that we need to associate with others – that we are members of a society – is utterly dependent on production, the satisfaction of material needs, and (historically) on the gradual increase in human population (Marx and Engels 1970: 51). Who we are, and those with whom we identify, presuppose how we make a living. Humans share a universal species being – or so Marx assumed, influenced by Enlightenment thought – but because what we do differs on a daily basis, we also fundamentally differ in how we think, feel and act.

Marx and Engels, prescient of so much anthropology to follow, did not expect the Inuit, for example, to resemble the Germans in their emotional, cognitive or social life. As Clifford Geertz (1973: 49) has famously said, 'there is no such thing as a human nature independent of culture. Men without culture … would be unworkable monstrosities with very few useful instincts, fewer recognizable sentiments, and no intellect: mental basket cases.' While this is an idealist har-monic on the Marxian theme, even Geertz recognises the import of what we do for who we are:

> To be human ... is not to be Everyman; it is to be a particular kind of man, and of course men differ. ... Within [Javanese]] society, differences are recognised, too – the way a rice peasant becomes human and Javanese differs from the way a civil servant does. (1973:53)

Although social identity – what it means to be a rice farmer – has received enormous attention over the years, the terms of the debate have shifted fundamentally during the last three decades. From an early Geertzian emphasis on the symbolic parameters of identity, the discussion moved first to the practices of identity and now to its bodily manifestations: that is, to how we act out our identities; indeed, how we bear them corporeally through sexuality, gender, comportment, the cultivation or modification of the body, clothing, and so on.

As Andrew Strathern and Michael Lambek (1998: 5) note with a certain humour, '[t]he body is suddenly omnipresent in academic texts'. In part, this is due to the 'increased visibility and objectification [of the body] within late capitalist consumer society'. Scholarly fascination with the body has been shaped as well by feminist critiques of essentialist views of sex and gender, and by 'the body's increased salience as primary signifier and locus of "home" for the uprooted, mobile, hybridized citizens of the transnational moment' (1998: 5). Concurrently, there is increased distrust of studying 'reified' cultural systems of identity, opting instead for the supposed certainties of practice, and the tangible evidence of embodiment. For a number of disciplines, imminence has become almost everything (Maynard 2002, 2003). Thus, the body, for Strathern and Lambek (1998: 5), is coming to replace the 'person' as a subject of inquiry, and I would add 'identity' as well.

For Strathern and Lambek, as well as Tamsin Wilton (1996), this signals a 'new materialism' in postmodernist thinking.[1]

> It is perhaps ironic that the anti-enlightenment tendency of postmodernism, with its suspicion of meta-narratives, its refusal to hierarchize truth-claims and its concomitant de-centring of science, has written the body back into theory. Ironic, because general opinion is that postmodernism is the ultimate in anti-materiality. ... Yet others insist that it is precisely the theoretical iconoclasm of postmodernism, the casting down of the throne of scientific rationalism, that enables the return of the body. (Wilton 1996: 102)

Circuitously, and paradoxically, we can return here to the insights of Marx and Engels, that consciousness and identity are rooted in our bodies and our work. Or, can we? Robert Ulin (2002: 692–3) reminds us of the long history of critique concerning Marx' concept of work – by Jürgen Habermas, Hannah Arendt, and others – who show how he conflates work with meeting utilitarian needs, at the expense of the cultural work by which we give meaning to what we do, and who we are.[2] For Habermas, especially, Marx focuses only on instrumentality, overlooking both the critical and communicative rationality of human beings. 'In short, instrumental views of work, and more generally human action, tend to eclipse, or at the very least to render derivative, social interaction as symbolic and the cultural construction of work and identity' (Ulin 2002: 693).

Taking French wine-growers as his example, Ulin examines how human agents construct their identity, but this work is not simply economic labour narrowly construed: it represents the full panoply of human activity. As such, it is grounded in interaction with others – with its implication of diverse cultural perspectives and unequal access to power – as well as the historical impedimenta and opportunities crucial to how we define both ourselves and our possibilities. As Ulin notes in the masthead above:

> [T]he culturally formative activity which is entailed in wine-growing work and identity unfolds in a social arena which positions wine-growers both literally and figuratively in fields of power and which should be seen as both historically and socially mediated. (2002: 694)

Put another way, work is inherently cultural. And, identity formation always implies – especially when it is part of larger culturalist movements – what Appadurai (1996: 15) calls 'the most general form of the work of the imagination'.

Working at medicine, imagining personhood

What does this mean for medical identity, and, more to the point, for the essays in this volume? If both our 'human nature' and our social identities are entwined with daily activities, then semi-specialities or occupations involved in medicine have a way of defining their practitioners. That is, if healers and other people engaged in medicine differ in what they do (and how they think of medicine, healing, and so on), then how they define themselves, and are defined by others, will likewise vary fundamentally. There may be, in fact, a world of difference between acupuncturists in China, diviners in South Africa, or care assistants in a British facility for the elderly. Even within the professional sector of biomedicine, medical identities may vary widely: consider here Jenny Littlewood's discussion of different interests and perspectives of midwives, nurses and obstetricians in a London hospital (p. 134). Finally, the same medical status may vary across time or in different social contexts. As Anne Digby demonstrates in her essay on physicians in Great Britain and South Africa (p. 14), the identities of general practitioners in rural Britain over the past century were often quite different from urban specialists, or their counterparts in the colonies.

Leslie Sharp (1993: 17) draws on Marcel Mauss (1987), along with Nancy Scheper-Hughes and Margaret Lock (1987), to set out the concept of 'the three bodies'; that is, we can distinguish three levels of identity: self, personhood and ethnic identity (or, in our case, medical identity). 'Selfhood', in this typology refers to the personal experience of identity, of who one is, though it is culturally shaped; personhood also pertains to the individual, but defines her 'as a social being who experiences *structural* shifts in relation to her kin and friends, and these shifts affect her role and status in the community' (Sharp 1993: 17, emphasis original). Ethnic identity, by contrast, focuses on the relation of the person (and self) to the group (1993: 17).

Though we can separate these concepts analytically, Sharp (1993: 17) under-scores their fluidity and dynamism. In her study of spirit possession in Madagas-car, as a medium enters and exits trance she may move between all three forms of identity, 'shifts that may be temporary or permanent.' Self, personhood and eth-nic or other social identities are cultural constructions, ineluctably tied to specific social circumstances. For example, we should be careful about associating the self too closely with either the individual or the body as presumably discrete 'things'. As Anne Becker (1995: 127) notes for the Fijians, 'Self-essence ... transcends the body to affiliate with the collective. The two, body and self, do not share a mutu-ally fixed or exclusive identity; their common substrate is the collective.'

From Richard Shweder and Edmund Bourne (1984: 193–4) we can conclude that the self and personhood – and certainly medical or other forms of social identity – vary cross-culturally, and are social constructs. Of course, the same is true in industrialised Western societies, so-called bastions of individualism. Here, too, the self is 'saturated' by, indeed relative to, social and cultural life (cf. Gergen 1991; Sennett 1998). Likewise, concepts of the self, person and identity vary over time; we certainly see that in Europe and North America (e.g., Sennett 1977; Tay-lor 1989; Reiss 2003), and we might expect to see it in non-Western nations and indigenous groups as well. In this light, we might consider the implications of cul-tural psychology, that the mind is culturally constituted (Cole 1996: 101f.).

The essays in this volume range across all three concepts – self, personhood, and social identity – to show their on-going dynamism and relation to practising medicine. All the authors underscore the keen observation of Maureen Schwarz (1997: 8), that 'over the last few decades, the classical anthropological opposition between the self – the awareness of oneself as a "perceptible object" (Hallowell 1955) – and the person as a social construct [and I would add social identity] has blurred'. Instead, these represent, in Gergen's deft phrase (1991: 156), 'relational realities.'

In this volume we see this fluidity most clearly in Gina Buijs' discussion of Zulu diviners (p. 84), especially men who receive female spirits and assume senses of self and personhood, bound up with transvestitism or homosexuality, that have profound implications for their social identities as diviners and healers. What does it mean for the individual 'male' *sangoma* to engage in such practices: how does it affect 'his' sense of self, 'his' prestige in the community, or even 'his' via-bility as a diviner?

We glimpse analogous questions in Elisabeth Hsu's distinction between 'par-ticipant observation' and 'participant experience' as she steered the latter course as an anthropologist, 'learning the skills and knowledge I intended to study to such a degree that I could perform these skills myself (p. 101)'. As her fascinating autobiographical account makes clear, there are profound implications for the self, personhood, and the larger social identity of the anthropologist in 'learning to be an acupuncturist, and not becoming one'.

The interweaving of self, personhood and social identity implies that who is recognised as having a medical identity, or who views themselves in this capacity, may vary over time. They may be thought of as quacks in one historical era, only to bear the imprimatur of authenticity in another. Or their legitimacy may never be in doubt, but their prestige may experience radical shifts in fortune. Such questions inform Anne Digby's discussion of rural British general practitioners. Her study likewise raises important methodological issues: rural GPs were often quite busy and not disposed culturally to record introspection about their medical identity. She poses the intriguing question: how does one study a group where self-effacement is part of their identity, where people assert that the 'private' self ought to be subsumed by 'public' experience?

We see a similar issue approached from a different vantage point by Jenny Littlewood in regard to midwife identity. When a birth goes wrong, or a baby is stillborn, what does it mean for the midwife's sense of self, as well as her personhood in relation to others, or her identity within the larger structures of the medical system and society? What are the implications for midwives of attempting to 're-naturalise' birth – to portray it as a highly personal, even intimate event between the mother, her partner and the baby – while also managing the birth technologically and bureaucratically?

Just as Littlewood situates the self and personhood of midwives in the context of their lower status and prestige relative to gynecologists, Janette Davies presents a similarly poignant structural dilemma for nursing-home care assistants: how do they conceive of themselves when they are essential to so much care-giving, yet are accorded such low social status and prestige (p. 117)? By 'conferring dignity' on patients, through the hard work of medical and personal care, auxiliary aides confer dignity on themselves. They see themselves as 'necessary go-betweens', with a profound sense of value that may outstrip the relatively menial sense of personhood accorded to them by nurses, administrators or, at times, the public.

If medical identity raises questions about society and the self, it also calls into question what we mean by 'medical'. That is, if the cultural work of identity points beyond mere utilitarian labour, as we have seen, then medicine, too, might imply a good deal more than biological or psychological health. Better said, medicine (again, as cultural work) has implications well beyond a narrow construal of healthcare as a material need for survival. Thus, I return to the adjective 'medical' in 'medical identity'. Medicine, as with most things, is defined in myriad ways cross-culturally. Indeed, in many indigenous societies medicine has far more to do with public welfare writ large than with solely interventive or preventive matters of illness (cf. Maynard 2004; Whyte 1997). As with the Kedjom of Cameroon in this volume (p. 61), health becomes only one diacritic amongst others denoting individual and social well-being; equally crucial may be economic prosperity, freedom from accidents, human fertility (as well as that of animals and plants), and indeed political sovereignty of the society. Likewise, how a practitioner approaches medicine – for example, as a ritual versus commercial act – may say volumes about the perceived authenticity of his or her identity. 'Commercial medicine' in societies like the Kedjom may be oxymoronic; healers who ask for cash on the barrelhead may risk charges of charlatanism.

Finally, all the essays in this volume situate identity, personhood and the self within the wider structures of society. If identity is culturally constructed, it may be shaped as well by class, gender, ethnicity, racism, sexuality, colonialism, the state, and other exogenous factors. Again, Anne Digby compares British GPs with their middle-class counterparts who emigrated to South Africa, and the latter with black South African physicians who came to Britain for their medical education. Finally, she considers how the emergence of state control of health care, through nationalization of the British health service after the Second World War, meant profound shifts in medical personhood. As members of the National Health Service, physicians assumed a profoundly different identity than the old self-employed rural practitioner.

Similar shifts are found in Cambodia, again in response to the state: in this case, the massive social experimentation imposed under the Khmer Rouge, followed by the contemporary impact of the transnational pharmaceutical industry and the dominance of neoliberal economic policies. For Ing-Britt Trankell and Jan Ovesen (p. 36), matters of identity are played out against two backdrops: cultural conceptions of modernity in regard to the assessment of medicines and their providers, as well as how various drug-providers position themselves in respect to distributing medicinal substances.

Just as identity is a relational reality, so, too, for Trankell and Ovesen, we can speak of the 'social lives of medicines'. But both medicine and our own social lives are deeply etched by underlying structural or transnational processes. Whether larger economic forces in Cambodia or Cameroon, sexuality in Zululand, class in Great Britain, or ethnicity in China, external factors help sculpt medical identity, how we conceive ourselves, and how others assess our status.

Working at medical identity: an order to the argument

Based on rich and diverse ethnographic data, the essays in this book look at the medical identity of a wide array of healers and other promoters of well-being – whether acupuncturists or physicians, diviners or nursing home providers, medicine sellers or midwives. The authors ask multiple questions: about the self-fashioning of medical personhood, how other people in the society view care-givers, or the degree to which wider social and cultural factors shape their medical identities. As I have said, these essays demonstrate that class, gender, sexuality, ethnicity, or state policy may all play formative roles in constructing definitions of health and well-being, how they are delivered, and the character and prestige of those who provide for our health and welfare in society.

As authors, we explicitly set out to consider multiple medical identities, in multiple social and cultural contexts, across historical eras, and at several analytic levels. From the interpersonal to the institutional, from fine-grained ethnographies of local realities to structural analyses of identity in the context of transnational forces, these essays underscore the sheer diversity of medical identities and the external factors that impinge upon them.

We begin with the apparently unproblematic – what might seem virtually iconic of 'medical identity' – and immediately begin to complicate it, namely, the identity of the general practitioner (GP) in Western biomedicine. Anne Digby works on multiple fronts to remind us that there is nothing natural, nothing inevitable about how physicians think about themselves, or what we assume about them. The GP's identity is both an historical construction, and cross-culturally variable. Indeed, it may not be the same in rural or urban areas, or in other contexts in the same society. Digby contrasts the social identity and self-image of rural practitioners with that of their urban counterparts; likewise, she demonstrates how they may differ from specialists in their cultural construction of self. Historically, rural GPs in Great Britain constructed a profoundly 'local' identity, one wedded to their involvement in the community, both professionally and socially. Just as they were 'general' practitioners, so too their identities were general, multifaceted and intricately interwoven with the community, across the lifespan, across generations, across all the most intimate, and most public, events that mark a specific place.

Digby complicates the picture still further. She shows us how rural medical identity has changed over the last century, from the Victorian era to the post-Second World War world of the National Health Service. We see, in particular, how larger demographic, economic, and political forces have helped transform the medical identity of rural GPs from an heroic, self-sacrificing image – influenced by a Romantic celebration of rural life fated to disappear – to the more professional, bureaucratic identity of a 'panel physician' within the National Health Service.

Digby goes on to illustrate how the identity of the GP has also changed under the impact of emigration, as physicians have left the UK, often for economic reasons, to practice in colonial South Africa. As representatives of the colonial power, practising in a different society and culture, in a situation dominated by a racist view of indigenous people, British physicians in South Africa have assumed a very different conception of themselves and their relationships with African patients, from that which they might assert in the Scottish Borders. Finally, Digby garners evidence to show how this process works in reverse, the impact on black physicians of leaving the rigid racist dichotomies of South Africa to receive medical education in Great Britain.

With the second chapter, we continue the analysis of Western biomedical identities, focusing more directly on the impact of other societies and cultures. Ing-Britt Trankell and Jan Ovesen consider the 'social life of medicine' in Cambodia, but rather than focus on physicians, they remind us of a major medical identity we may often forget: the pharmacist, chemist or local drug-providers. They consider two major macro-level external influences on such identities: the rise and aftermath of the Khmer Rouge regime and the advent of Western pharmaceutical transnational corporations in the Cambodian market. Drawing on a distinction by Vinh-Kim Nguyen and Karine Peschard (2003), Trankell and Ovesen argue that medical identity is shaped by three orientations in Cambodia: premodern, modern and a-modern (rather than 'postmodern') medical views. The premodern orientation of indigenous herbalists merges healing and curing, whereas the modernist view of the professional pharmacist focuses principally on curing biological pathologies through a capitalist exchange, the purchase of bio-medicine. The vast majority of the population, however, and most of the commercial chemists, dwell more in an a-modern medical world, one that merges capitalist and indigenous assumptions in the same transaction.

In the third chapter on so-called 'traditional doctors', Kent Maynard charts similar terrain in Cameroon, though he focuses more intently on local forms of medicine. For the Kedjom people, we see a new tradition of healers, arising essentially since the Second World War, merging the iconography and etiology of the precolonial medicinal sphere with the principles of commercial exchange and Western institutional arrangements of hospital care. As with many medicine sellers in Cambodia, Kedjom 'traditional doctors' forge uneasy relationships between the precolonial and modernist principles of local and biomedicine. The question is: how do potential clients respond to their claims to a new medical identity? Maynard argues that patients are pragmatic yet cautious. They may go to such healers, and end up valorizing their assumptions about the practice of medicine for profit, if and only if healers are successful. Yet, if the therapeutic process fails they may become disenchanted, wondering if the healer has exaggerated his or her power for the sake of money. As a result, the trajectory of many healers can be meteoric; they may become immensely popular, but their success may be short-lived indeed.

Again for sub-Saharan Africa, but this time for diviners, Gina Buijs asks a question similar to Maynard's: how do potential clients respond to the identity claims of practitioners? In Buijs' case study, drawn from South Africa, this question is complicated less by what happens in Kedjom – turning medicine into a commercial transaction – than by the sexual orientation of the diviner. What do Zulu laypersons say about diviners, supposedly celibate, who may engage in homosexual practices? Interestingly enough, very few such diviners are denied legitimacy. In Buijs' account we see both how such diviners may construct their ambiguous sexual and gender identities, and the social and cultural context that allows them to continue practising as diviners.

Buijs is able to accomplish several matters in this chapter. On the one hand, she makes the important ethnographic point that homosexuality and transvestism are more institutionalised in sub-Saharan Africa than we might think. She makes an equally important point about why it may be condoned, if not accepted, that it does not de-legitimise the identity of the diviner. While transvestism is practised quite openly, homosexual relationships are not. They may be 'public secrets', that is, known at some level by everyone, yet never subjected so glaringly to scrutiny that such practices call into question the other identities of the person. This is due in part, Buijs observes, to the power of the diviner: they enjoy genuine cultural legitimacy in regard to their role as diviners, an authority that may override other aspects of their identity that might otherwise cause them to be stigmatised.

In Elisabeth Hsu's chapter, 'Learning to be an acupuncturist, and not becoming one', she considers a new region of the world and a new medical identity – acupuncturists in China – but also a somewhat different question that we have asked before. That is, she asks simultaneously about the identities of acupuncturists and her own as an anthropologist. Concurrently, she poses a methodological question that connects them: how can she best learn what it is like to be acupuncturist? For Hsu the answer lies in her distinction between 'participant observation' and 'participant experience'. She opts for the latter as both more humane and more methodologically sound: 'Engaging in participant experience meant to me that I should be involved learning the skills and knowledge I intended to study to such a degree that I could perform those skills myself'. Hsu's chapter, as a result, wends a distinctive path, a double journey as it turns out, exploring both what it means to be an acupuncturist and what it is like to become one as an anthropologist. Again, what we learn about the former (and the latter), as with all medical identities, is that they are shaped fundamentally by larger structural and institutional factors, both internal and external to medicine. For acupuncturists we see how they lack the prestige of doctors who practice Chinese classical medicine. But Hsu also shows us how their conceptions of the body, of *loci* and channels, bear the imprint of deep cultural roots, a set of widely shared cultural assumptions that may lend credence to the legitimacy of their identity.

In Janette Davies's chapter we return to the West, but to care assistants in a nursing home especially for those suffering various forms of dementia. Yet, as with acupuncturists in China, care givers in the UK must contend with a lower status in the medical hierarchy. Davies shows us tellingly the impact of a paradox on their identity: on the one hand they are considered virtually 'menial workers' in the wider reward system of biomedicine, yet on the other they are absolutely crucial to care within the residential home. Highly valuable yet undervalued; in such circumstances how do caregivers conceive their medical identity? Auxiliary workers, most of whom are women, draw on another of their identities – that of mother, wife or daughter – to give care where care is needed. By doing so, they affirm that what they do is essential, in spite of its low prestige and compensation. Although they occupy a world of commodified labour, they view what they do less as work than as care. Thus, by conceptually removing themselves from the commercial sphere and reconfiguring who they are more in the domestic arena, they attribute to themselves a value beyond price.

It is intriguing, and no accident, that similar themes emerge in Jenny Littlewood's final chapter, on midwives in a London hospital. She, too, demonstrates where midwives fit in the wider biomedical hierarchy, how their lower status and prestige contribute to their attempts to professionalise their identity as important to the birthing process. For Littlewood, this produces its own share of ironies: although midwives have gained prestige and status in professional medicine, they have done so at the expense of reducing their role in the community. As with Digby's discussion of rural physicians in Great Britain who joined the National Health Service (NHS); their identity has shifted from a local focus to a national one, their identification with the lay community has now shifted more to professional colleagues.

Yet, Littlewood equally shows us that the trauma of a less than 'perfect' birth may leave the midwife on her own, bereft of potential ties with either the community or her colleagues. We see here another irony: much of the midwife's sense of self and identity is premised on personal, hands-on involvement in facilitating a 'normal' birth. The midwife helps to construct this event as a natural, intimate event shared between her, the mother, her partner, and the newborn baby. Yet, this takes place within a highly bureaucratic, technological setting, one structured by the NHS to maximize statistics on 'successful' pregnancies. Midwives must, in effect, bridge contradictory cultural constructions: the personal and the bureaucratic, the natural and the technological, the intimate and the impersonal. This implies an inherently risky process of identification and selfhood, and Littlewood shows us clearly that there may be real 'costs' involved in the achievement of 'normal births.'

Conclusions

In the end, we are who we are through hard work. Work never done alone, but always with a profound sense of agency (the power to make a difference), is underscored by all the essays in this volume. Sometimes the work of medical identity is quite conscious – a matter of self-invention; more often, our identity emerges unbidden out of experience. What that experience is, the specific contours of the work, and how it bears the brunt of larger cultural and social matters, shape what we do and what we think about it. Working at or working in medicine is not unproblematic: the work itself, what we mean by medicine, and how it makes us (and others) feel about who we are, are all matters to be discovered. As these essays demonstrate, where the cultural work of medical identity ends up is equally something to be investigated, not assumed.

Notes

1. Terence Turner (1994: 30) introduces a perceptive note of caution about the tenuousness of this materialism, at least in post-structuralism:

> The elevation of the body to the place occupied by subject, agent and social individual in older forms of Western social thought, notwithstanding its apparently 'materialist' character as a substitution of a concrete physical entity for an abstract metaphysical concept, has generally involved in practice a focus on conceptual or linguistic representations of the body and an indifference to the body as an objective physical reality.

Thus, post-structuralists (and postmodernists) may hypothetically get us back to the body – as I imply in the next paragraph – but we need to complete important conceptual work to understand the body in all its senses, cognition and corporality, as an agent in the fullest sense, not simply as a semiotic text inscribed passively by culture (or Foucault's 'power/knowledge'), and read by someone else.

2. I am grateful to Jenny Littlewood in her chapter for this volume, reminding me of Ulin's (2002) trenchant essay on French wine-growers and their cultural work in constructing identity.

References

Appadurai, A. 1996. *Modernity at Large: Cultural Dimensions of Globalization*. Minneapolis: University of Minnesota Press.

Becker, A.E. 1995. *Body, Self, and Society: The View from Fiji*. Philadelphia: University of Pennsylvania Press.

Boddy, J. 1989. *Wombs and Alien Spirits: Women, Men, and the Zar Cult in Northern Sudan*. Madison: University of Wisconsin Press.

Cole, M. 1996. *Cultural Psychology: A Once and Future Discipline*. Cambridge: Belknap Press of Harvard University Press.

Comaroff, J. 1994. 'Defying Disenchantment: Reflections on Ritual, Power, and History'. In *Asian Visions of Authority: Religion and the Modern States of East and Southeast Asia*. C.F. Keyes, L. Kendall and H. Hardacre (eds), Honolulu: University of Hawaii Press.

Corin, E. 1998. 'Refiguring the Person: The Dynamics of Affects and Symbols in an African Spirit Possession Cult'. In *Bodies and Persons: Comparative Perspectives from Africa and Melanesia*. M. Lambek and A. Strathern (eds), Cambridge: Cambridge University Press.

Geertz, C. 1973. *The Interpretation of Cultures: Selected Essays*. New York: Basic Books.

Gergen, K.J. 1991. *The Saturated Self: Dilemmas of Identity in Contemporary Life*. New York: Basic Books.

Hallowell, H.I. 1955. *Culture and Experience*. Philadelphia: University of Pennsylvania Press.

Lan, D. 1985. *Guns and Rain: Guerillas and Spirit Mediums in Zimbabwe*. London: James Currey.

Marx, K. and F. Engels. 1970. *The German Ideology*. Part 1. Ed. C.J. Arthur. London: Lawrence and Wishart.

Masquelier, A. 2001. *Prayer Has Spoiled Everything: Possession, Power, and Identity in an Islamic Town of Niger*. Durham, NC: Duke University Press.

Mauss, M. 1987. 'A Category of the Human Mind: The Notion of the Person; the Notion of the Self'. In *The Category of the Person: Anthropology, Philosophy, and History*. M. Carrithers, S., Collins and S. Lukes (eds), Cambridge: Cambridge University Press.

Maynard, K. 2002. 'An "Imagination of Order": The Suspicion of Structure in Anthropology and Poetry'. *Antioch Review* 60(20: 220–43.

———— 2003. 'Thirteen Ways of Looking at a Camel'. *Anthropology News* 44(2): 8 and 11.

———— 2004. *Making Kedjam Medicine: A History of Public Health and Well-Being in Cameroon*. Westport, CT: Praeger.

Nguyen, V-K. and K. Peschard. 2003. 'Anthropology, Inequality and Disease: A Review'. *Annual Review of Anthropology* 32: 447–74.

Rasmussen, S. 1995. *Spirit Possession and Personhood Among the Kel Ewey Tuareg*. Cambridge: Cambridge University Press.

Reiss, T.J. 2003. *Mirages of the Self: Patterns of Personhood in Ancient and Early Modern Europe*. Stanford: Stanford University Press.

Scheper-Hughes, N. and M. Lock. 1987. 'The Mindful Body: A Prolegomenon to Future Work in Medical Anthropology'. *Medical Anthropology Quarterly* 1(1): 1–36.

Schwarz, M. 1997. *Molded in the Image of Changing Woman: Navajo Views on the Human Body and Personhood*. Tucson: University of Arizona Press.

Sennett, R. 1977. *The Fall of Public Man*. New York: Knopf.

———— 1998. *The Corrosion of Character: The Personal Consequences of Work in the New Capitalism*. New York: W.W. Norton.

Sharp, L.A. 1993. *The Possessed and the Dispossessed: Spirits, Identity, and Power in a Madagascar Migrant Town*. Berkeley: University of California Press.

Shaw, R. 2002. *Memories of the Slave Trade: Ritual and the Historical Imagination in Sierra Leone*. Chicago: University of Chicago Press.

Shweder, R.A. and E.J. Bourne. 1984. 'Does the Concept of the Person Vary Cross-Culturally?' In *Culture Theory: Essays on Mind, Self, and Emotion*. R.A. Shweder and R.A. LeVine (ed), Cambridge: Cambridge University Press.

Strathern, A. and M. Lambek. 1998. 'Introduction Embodying Sociality: Africanist – Melanesianist Comparisons'. In *Bodies and Persons: Comparative Perspectives from Africa and Melanesia*. M. Lambek and A. Strathern (eds), Cambridge: Cambridge University Press.

Taylor, C. 1989. *Sources of the Self: The Making of the Modern Identity*. Cambridge: Harvard University Press.

Turner, T. 1994. 'Bodies and Anti-bodies: Flesh and Fetish in Contemporary Social Theory'. In *Embodiment and Experience: The Existential Ground of Culture and Self*. T. Csordas (ed.), Cambridge: Cambridge University Press.

Ulin, R.C. 2002. 'Work as Cultural Production: Labour and Self-Identity Among Southwest French Wine-Growers'. *Journal of the Royal Anthropological Institute* 8: 691–712.

Whyte, S.R. 1997. *Questioning Misfortune: The Pragmatics of Uncertainty in Eastern Uganda*. Cambridge: Cambridge University Press.

Wilton, T. 1996. 'Genital Identities: An Idiosyncratic Foray into the Gendering of Sexualities'. In *Sexualizing the Social: Power and the Organization of Sexuality*. L. Adkins and V. Merchant (eds), New York: St Martin's.

1

SHAPING NEW IDENTITIES: GENERAL PRACTITIONERS IN BRITAIN AND SOUTH AFRICA

Anne Digby

The humanities and social sciences have seen a surge of interest in the topic of identity during recent decades, with the adoption of varied approaches from the structural to the phenomenological (Castells 1997; Craib 1998; Jenkins 1996; Rutherford 1990a; Woodward 1997). This chapter follows Rosen in 'taking the social character of medicine as a point of departure' and utilises mainly, but not exclusively, a social constructionist approach to explore the multiplicity of identities of general practitioners (Rosen 1967: 5–23). It discusses both the historical specificities and diverse dimensions of medical identities in providing an overview of the British general practitioner (GP) from the mid-nineteenth to mid-twentieth centuries. In addition, a briefer characterisation of the related history of the generalist in South Africa is included, in order to highlight the ways in which identities may be challenged and defined by difference.

The period covered in this chapter is marked by a number of important professional watersheds. For the British medical profession, the Medical Act of 1858 marked the beginning of modern general practice by laying down standards of training and of qualification, and requiring state registration of the qualified doctor, thus constructing some central identifying characteristics of the members of a profession. Two other structural changes shaped the identities of the modern British generalist – the National Health Insurance Act of 1911 and the National Health Service Act of 1946 – both of which enabled the doctor to treat a larger proportion of the population. The former initiated a state social insurance scheme for poorer patients whereby GPs could elect to go on a 'panel' to treat patients, and would receive some public money by doing so, whilst at the same time retaining the freedom to run a private practice. And in 1948 a comprehensive, National Health Service was implemented, through which all citizens could obtain treatment free at the point of access.

In contrast with Britain, organised medicine in South Africa had fewer professional disjunctures. Licensing of duly qualified practitioners by a central Colonial Medical Council or Committee dated from 1807, the year after the Cape Colony became a British territory, and continued thereafter with relatively minor modifications in 1891 and 1928. Licensing was based on a doctor having European qualifications, overwhelmingly British ones, until this was supplemented from the 1920s by doctors with qualifications gained from a training in South Africa. Conspicuous racial diversity in South Africa meant that doctors had a more heterogeneous cultural identity than those in Britain. There were two major racial sub-sets amongst white doctors – Afrikaners (of Dutch, German or French descent) and British – as well as a later, smaller group of black doctors (African, Indian, and 'Coloured'.)

The political union of the four South African provinces in 1910 brought together larger groups of doctors having a predominantly 'British' allegiance in the Cape and Natal, with the smaller, mainly Afrikaner medical groups in the Orange Free State and the Transvaal. Ensuing strains then meant that it was not until 1926 that agreement was reached to have a common association and journal for all South African doctors. Before this, Afrikaner medics as an organised group had stood somewhat aloof from British ones, disliking the imperial connection so conspicuous in a professional organisation based on Branches of the British Medical Association, an imperial organisation with one-fifth of its members resident in the overseas British Empire (Johnson and Caygill 1972–3: 304). Professional tensions between the South African organisation and the London-centred British Medical Association continued, although it was not until after the Second World War that the South African medical profession severed its ties, thus becoming the first of the British Medical Association's imperial Branches to become autonomous. In this rupture of loyalties the medical profession effectively anticipated the South African government's move in 1961 to independent political status as a Republic (Johnson and Caygill 1972–3: 321–3).

Within this framework of common, if by no means uncontested, political and professional affiliations, the medical professions within the two countries had both similarities and dissimilarities. In 1948 there were an estimated 17,600 general practitioners in England and Wales, and a further 2,000 in Scotland. In a country that was geographically four times as large, South Africa had a much smaller number: only 4,784 doctors had trained in Western medicine by that date (Webster 1988: 122; Oosthuizen 1957: 289–91). But both countries had largely male medical professions: in Britain by the 1930s only one in ten members of the profession was a woman, a position reached slightly later during the 1960s in South Africa (Walker 2001: 484, 487, 490, 493–5, 498–500; Digby 1999: 161–2). Whereas the average doctor-population ratio in South Africa was one doctor to 1,681 people in 1948, in Britain at the same date the ratio was less than half this, with one doctor to only 813 people (*SAMJ* 1957: 290–1).

In each country there were conspicuous regional and local disparities in these ratios, more particularly between 'under-doctored' rural areas and urban practices with much more favourable ratios. Rapid British urbanisation meant that the one in two rural inhabitants of the mid-nineteenth century had been reduced to only one in five by the early twentieth century. By this time, the small number of rural patients and the high travelling expenses involved in reaching them – together with the tendency of some suburban doctors to use their cars to invade the practice areas of their rural colleagues – was even beginning to threaten the survival of the British country doctor. Under the National Health Insurance scheme of 1911 the state increasingly recognised the financial difficulties of these practitioners by providing subsidies for their practices. This was necessary to offset the attractions of urban practice. Here the ambitious generalist, exploiting greater professional opportunities for more diversified practice with better access to hospitals, could develop a practice with a higher income potential.

In the much more rural territory of South Africa the census of 1911 showed a not dissimilar distribution of doctors with medical practitioners crowded in the large towns, so that only a minority of doctors worked in the country's vast rural interior, varying from one in ten of the profession in the Cape Province to one in three in Natal (Union of South Africa Parliamentary Papers: 706–7). However, in later years there was a gradual increase in the proportion of the profession who worked outside the large towns (*SAMJ* 1957: 290–1). Even so, rural areas with large black populations continued to have very few doctors, not least because practitioners did not think they could make an adequate medical living in these areas.

The vast majority of those practising medicine in both countries were GPs, but it was the specialists who increasingly dominated the medical profession: medical training was dictated by their needs, and reputation was geared to success in specialism, not general practice. It was the specialists whose autobiographies, biographies and obituaries defined the peaks of professional success and shaped the images of modern medicine. The identities of the 'footsoldiers' (the GPs) rather than the 'generals' (the specialists and consultants) of the medical profession are less easy to discover. As one British obituary aptly remarked: 'I should like to pay tribute to this really great general practitioner. He is one of the many "Unknown Soldiers" who form the backbone of the medical profession' (*BMJ* 1941: 178).[1] One example of this group was Dr Huskie, who on his retirement told his patients on the Scottish Borders that:

> He had now been at it for 52 years. At his old university of Edinburgh it had been impressed upon him that his first duty was self-effacement; his work in the first place was to relieve suffering, the first thing was the good of his patients, and [he was] at all times to keep himself in the background and to keep in touch with progress in his profession. He had tried to carry out these ideals to the best of his ability. (*Moffat News*, 8 August 1940)

The personal and private identities of people who practise self-effacement are not necessarily easy to construct, so that some potentially interesting questions cannot be pursued because of lack of evidence, although for other issues a variety of sources and approaches permit us to interrogate the identities of general practitioners in Britain and South Africa to gain fresh insights.

Cultural representations of British identity

To introduce the subject a variety of literary and artistic images before and after the watershed Medical Act of 1858 are used to access cultural images of the British generalist. Two mid-nineteenth-century literary representations of the GP reveal much about their evolving position in society as well as their popular stereotyping. George Eliot's *Middlemarch: A Study of Provincial Life* was written in 1870–1 but depicted England in the years before the Great Reform Act of 1832, and was a study of social and political change as reflected in the histories of the characters. The novel provides an interesting depiction of medicine before the professional transformations involved in the 1858 act, notably through the characterisation of Dr Lydgate whose ambition to become a clinician was frustrated by the materialism inherent in an ill-judged marriage, so that perforce he became a fashionable doctor, whose economic success was heavily qualified by regret about lost professional aspiration. Lydgate had come from a well-connected Northumberland family, and Eliot shows how the ladies of the county were puzzled by his uncertain status as a country doctor, and wondered whether he should be identified as a gentleman or not. Lady Chettam mused about Lydgate's birth: 'One does not expect it in a practitioner of that kind, For my own part, I like a medical man more on a footing with the servants, they are oftener all the cleverer' (Eliot 1996: 84). This highlighted the social ambiguity of the medical man in a transitional era when advancing professionalisation was cutting across accepted status markers of birth and inherited gentility.

A study of another fictional GP, the Barsetshire *Dr Thorne* (1858), was so successful that Trollope, considered it 'the most popular book I have ever written'. In this novel Dr Thorne is shown as being criticised by his colleagues, who looked down on his tradesman-like dispensing of his own medicines, but disliked even more his publication of his charges – seven shillings and sixpence within a circuit of seven miles and more for longer distances. Trollope wrote that:

> A physician should take his fee without letting his left hand know what his right hand was doing; it should be taken without a thought, without a look, without a move of the facial muscles; the true physician should hardly be aware that the last friendly grasp of the hand had been made more precious by the touch of gold. Whereas that fellow Thorne would lug out half a crown from his breeches pocket and give it in change for a ten-shilling piece. (Trollope 1980: xi, 32–3)

Here his colleagues disliked the way Dr Thorne was continuing earlier practices of charging for the commodity of medicine like any trader in patent medicines, instead of adopting newer professional procedures by which the modern doctor charged for his skilled attendance. Rather than providing a handwritten bill of itemised pills and medicines, the up-to-date doctor was sending out a printed bill stating that s/he was charging so many guineas 'for professional services' (Digby 1994: 150–1).

These literary images may usefully be supplemented by two late Victorian portraits, both painted after the Medical Act, and perhaps because of this, each suggesting a greater professional dignity and *gravitas*. A painting of 1888 called simply *Duty*, gives us a respectful perspective of the public face of the country doctor as a dedicated professional in a portrayal more realistic than romaticised, although a possible Romantic reading might equate the natural background with the health that this medical professional was seeking to promote (reproduced in Wood 1988: 117 and Wallen 2004: 5). Heywood Hardy depicted an elderly doctor, asking directions from a shepherd boy as to how to get to a remote patient, and showed the doctor riding across a wild, barren landscape under a lowering sky. The viewer might reflect that the cost to the doctor in terms of time and energy was unlikely to be recouped from the patient's fee, and that the practitioner must have been well aware that this was the case, yet his obligation to minister to the needs of the sick gave him no alternative. The sombre colours of the portrait provide a concrete rendering of the bleakness of the GP's professional scenario.

Luke Fildes' more famous painting of 1891, *The Doctor* (Tate, London), showed a more nuanced fusion of the public and private face than had Hardy. Fildes attempted to depict more directly the practitioner's personal feelings within a professional encounter by painting an obviously preoccupied doctor gazing with sympathetic concern at a dying child in impoverished surroundings. It is clear that the limited therapeutic competence of the traditional doctor is inadequate to save the patient (Fildes 1968). Equally obvious is the fact that he was devoting plentiful time even to a poverty-stricken family that is unlikely to be able to recompense him.

How do these cultural representations relate to the professional lives and identities of GPs? Do they shape as well as reflect their characters? To a substantial extent I think that these images did mirror the qualities and features of the GP. For example, a country doctor like Dr David Huskie could well have been a model for Heywood Hardy's artistic portrait of '*Duty*.' He had a practice area in Lowland Scotland that stretched from his base in Moffat some 23 miles into Selkirkshire, and the same distance into Lanarkshire, as well as 20 miles into Peebleshire. Beginning practice in 1891, he recollected at the end of his working years that:

> It has been a hard and strenuous life, and for years I seldom got to my bed on the same day that I left it; and frequently two or three nights in the week I never got to bed at all - arriving home only in time to have a bath and breakfast and start my rounds again ... Still the life had its compensations. They were a kindly and grateful folk to work amongst, and very many of them staunch and loyal friends. (Huskie 1938: 12)[2]

As Britain became an increasingly urbanised country, doctors like Dr Huskie became a minority of the profession even, as we have seen, part of a financially –threatened sector. By the late nineteenth century, when the harsh legacy of earlier rapid industrialisation was being revealed in contemporary poverty surveys, a vanishing rural past became romanticised as part of an earlier golden age. Like other features of the dwindling rural scene, the country doctor tended increasingly to be placed within a sunset haze of affectionate nostalgia, as can see be seen from the conspicuous success of a later, long-running television series. 'Dr Finlay's Casebook' re-enacted the largely vanished world of a small Scottish community in which a well-known, respected family doctor delivered generations of babies and held the medical histories of local families in his head. In reality it was largely in the Scottish Highlands and Scottish Borders, as well as in the hill country of north Wales or northern England, that country doctors like this survived to win high status and esteem from their work in small, patient-centred practices.[3]

While Heywood Hardie's graphic depiction of this resilient breed of rural stalwart is almost entirely unknown, Fildes' painting is amongst the most familiar images of the general practitioner. Hardie's doctor is an almost abstract representation of duty, while Fildes' doctor is portrayed in a heroic, personalised and prolonged struggle with death, through the practitioner's vain attempts to save a sick child. The doctor is based on an actual historical figure, Dr Murray, the family doctor who had failed to save the artist's desperately ill child some years earlier. Fildes' picture became an extremely popular painting within the profession: British medical schools displayed it prominently, the American Medical Association selected it for the commemorative stamp of its centenary year, and British doctors chose to hang it in their waiting rooms. By promoting such an idealised image to the public, doctors may have been attempting to offset the reality of occupational commercialism by an image of disinterested professionalism. That this was probably done unconsciously is indicated by the fact that generations of GPs identified so readily with the image.

Identity is composed both of exclusion and of inclusion. The portrait excluded the pressures of commerce, and the inconvenient fact that time was money for the hard-pressed doctor, while it included – indeed, made prominent – the implications of the Hippocratic Oath for doctors' duty to do their utmost for their patients' health. Fildes' blend of the authentic and the idealised appealed strongly to the general practitioner's self-image, and arguably even helped shape self-identity through its ideal depiction of professional honour, exertion and responsibility.[4] Medical culture thus invested the image with layers of meaning that reconstituted the professional viewer through cultural points of identification. Indeed, a leader of the medical profession advised medical students about to start their careers to 'remember always to hold before you the ideal figure of Luke Fildes' picture, and be at once gentle men and gentle doctors' (quoted in Fildes 1968: 118).

Aspirations and realities in Britain

Medical school helped individuals internalise a medical culture and so construct a professional identity, not least by supplying role models of how doctors might present themselves to the world, providing templates for how things should be done, and indicating how situations could be tackled without losing face. Medical training has helped institutionalise identity by constructing a collective professional persona, with habitualised ways of seeing, patterns of behaviour and routines of activity.[5] It also altered the experiential world of young aspirant clinicians by changing their perceptions in learning how to construct patients' bodies as objects of diagnosis and therapy (Good 1994: 65–6, 72). At the end of successful training British professional qualifications gave objective markers of identity by conferring the ability to be admitted to the *Medical Register*, and hence to hold public appointments. During training general practitioner identities were shaped both by the similitude of collective identity in a common medical culture, and also by differentiation through the creation of a medical hierarchy where high fliers would become specialists, and the remaining three-quarters would go into general practice. Levels of identity were also later differentiated: whereas the specialist sought national or international recognition, the generalist made a professional investment in a local community, which then acknowledged this through appreciative respect.

The varied lifestyles which doctors wished to live, as well as the interface between public and private in the lives of doctors, were not well documented historically, precisely because many doctors lived such busy lives that they did not have enough time to write up the case histories of their patients, let alone to reflect on their own lives. There are few autobiographies that embody the self in narrative, thereby supplying valuable clues on the construction of identity, or evaluating its overlapping dimensions (Goffman 1974). Those that were written were less a matter of reflexifity, and hence of pondering about a lifetime's construction of the self, than an empirical, outwardly objective account of professional practice. The dynamic interaction between internal and external stimuli was not usually made explicit, so that the attitudes and feelings of the central figure were largely a matter of inference by the reader. The unspoken message of the genre was that generalists were concerned with what they did rather than who they were. That a private self was subsumed by public experience was evident in titles such as James Mullin's *A Toiler's Life* (1921), W. Robinson's *Sidelights on the Life of a Wearside Surgeon* (1939), C. B. Gunn's *Leaves from the Life of a Country Doctor* (1947), or H. W. Pooler's *My Life in General Practice* (1948). Only a few individuals were more open about their subjective motivation or their psychological reactions to professional experience (Huskie 1938; Jalland 1989). In contrast, the few biographies of pioneering medical women gave unusual prominence to their subjects' attitudes towards their profession by highlighting emotional feelings about topics such as the personal price paid for an onerous lifestyle, or discussing the character of distinctive relationships with female and child patients (Malleson 1919; St John 1935).

The relationship between doctors and their patients was an important feature of professional identity. A major source of information on this was the obituary, which gave standardised information on doctors' lives. Given constraints on length, an obituarist's selection of information gives an insight into the ways in which doctors wished to be remembered, and hence into the elements they thought of particular importance in professional identities. Following details of professional training, practice location and appointments, qualifications, clinical achievements, honours, and public recognition, came other information including some on relationships with local communities, and with patients. Personal qualities such as sympathy, kindness, and generosity were frequently cited as important in patient-doctor relationships, as were certain professional attributes such as painstaking attention or scrupulous care.

For a less anodyne discussion, however, sources on the small minority of female GPs are more illuminating because they are more detailed. For early medical women the desire to serve other women had been an imperative in their decision to enter medicine. 'My dream ... is that it will be looked on as one of the barbarisms of a past age that a medical man should ever have attended a woman' stated Mary Murdoch (quoted in Malleson 1919: 178). For female patients to be able to consult a practitioner of their own sex had fuelled their vocational choice, and continued to be paramount in their relationships with patients in practices which typically were made up of women and child clients (Digby 1999: 164, 172). At her death in 1923 Caroline O'Connor was said to have received 'many ill-spelt touching letters sent by individual working women who had crowded her surgery. "She never thought of herself, we all feel we have lost a friend."'[6] Identifying with these patients as fellow women, female GPs committed huge amounts of energy and time to them, sacrificing much hope of private life to their professional priority in realising a whole-hearted client-centred approach. Mary Murdoch recognised without regret that medicine had been 'an exacting mistress, and has taken thing after thing away from me; tethered me down, taken my freedom and liberty'. And Margaret Norton stated that: 'I never was ruled by the clock ... people are all so different, and this is what's ... such fun about general practice. This is what's made the whole life' (Malleson 1919: 37).[7]

Tensions between professional aspirations and realities, as well as between private and public needs, can be discerned in sale advertisements of generalists' practices. Advertisements of good practices were grounded in reality for a minority of fortunate individuals, but at the same time highlighted the kind of lives that many more of their colleagues might have wished to achieve. These were less grandiose dreams of ideal medical landscapes to explore than aspirations that might be possible if fortune smiled on them (Anderson 1983). The problem of generalising about a very diverse set of lifestyles within the medical profession is clearly illustrated by two Edwardian advertisements of contrasting practices. The first combined utopian and practical elements in promising for an affluent doctor an attractive, but professionally unusual, life of a leisured gentleman with few pressures:

Cathedral City – Nice practice of about £450 a year. Unlimited scope. Good house, specially built, every modern convenience ... Golf (10 minutes), tennis, boating, fishing, shooting, hunting and polo, all handy. No carriage required. Night work declined and midwifery discouraged ... The house is situated in the best residential part.

A contrasting advertisement appeared soon afterwards: 'For disposal – surgery only been open 3 months. At present doing little but good opening for a man who can afford to wait a little time. It is situated in a thickly populated working class suburb of Manchester' (*BMJ* Supplement, 2 October and 2 December 1909). This advertisement for a marginal practice was not unusual at this time when, within a crowded medical market, one in ten doctors earned less than £300 gross per annum, and a further one in ten between £300 and £400 (Digby 1994: table 5.2). Unlike their more established colleagues, these struggling practitioners had to assume the spurious appearance of busy professional activity in order to try to attract a few patients.

Migration and the shaping of new identities in South Africa

The desire of the Victorian middle class for their children to enter the professions meant that these became increasingly overcrowded in Western Europe (Digby 1999: 23–9). As a result, Britain's medical schools produced too many doctors for available openings, so that young doctors were forced to shape new livelihoods for themselves. One important avenue – particularly evident during the 1880s and 1890s, and again during the interwar years – was emigration to less professionally crowded lands in the British Empire. The Cape Province in South Africa was quite a popular destination, not least because discoveries of diamonds and gold in the 1870s and 1880s provided a 'pull' factor so that it appeared, misleadingly in terms of its economic reality, as a virtual 'Medical El Dorado' (Digby 1995: 464–79).

As a British colony the Cape's system of medical licensing privileged those with British medical qualifications, and more than nine out of ten of those licensed to practice in the Cape between 1810 and 1910 had qualified in Britain (Phillips 2004). The President of the Western Cape's Medical Association remarked in 1888 that 'The great majority of practitioners out here are all, in one way or other, associated with the older universities and colleges of the Mother Country, and it is a source of great pleasure and interest to us all, to cherish the best "traditions" and practice of our profession as handed down to us' (Dr C.K. Murray, BMA Presidential Addresses, 1908: 2–3). The long-established white settler population and the healthiness of the temperate Cape meant that its relational identity with Britain was one of substantial similarity, having a degree of 'foreignness' much less than in tropical African regions (often perceived as the 'white man's grave') which were interpreted as helping to shape a British identity through their colonial 'otherness' (Bewell 1999: 18).

The close ties created between the Cape and British medical professions facilitated entry by British medical migrants, whether these were impoverished practitioners seeking to make a medical living, sick doctors in search of a healthier
climate, or missionaries hoping to use medical skills to convert their patients.
Nevertheless, a very different colonial situation forged new attitudes and skills
among medical emigrants, creating novel identities in the process. The Cape's ear-
liest female doctor, a former missionary, illustrated this. Jane Waterston
(1843–1932) preferred the challenges of the Cape to her homeland of Scotland.
'Civilisation bores me, and luxury does not suit me. I seem made for a younger
country and a simpler life,' she wrote.[8] Rutherford has aptly commented on this
process: 'Identification ... is an interchange between self and structure, a transforming process' (Rutherford 1990b: 14).

Some young Scottish or Irish-trained graduates who had little chance of making a viable medical living in their home country accepted government posts as
Cape district surgeons, seeing them as a useful initial stage in creating a new life
and constructing a livelihood based on a public salaried appointment together
with a private general practice. The government post involved treating mainly
impoverished patients of whom the majority were black, whereas most of the private patients were likely to have been white. Since in rural areas many doctors
would have held such a public appointment, little status differentiation was evident between them.

In May 1895 John McIver wrote to introduce himself to the colonial
administration in Cape Town: 'I am 25 years of age, about 5ft 10 in height, a
graduate of Edinburgh University and a Scotchman.' He enclosed testimonials
from his teachers, one of whom mentioned that ill health had precluded him
from completing his course. MacIver himself soon made it clear that the state of
his health meant that he needed a post in an elevated, dry situation.[9] He was
appointed as the District Surgeon to Sutherland, and was based in Clanwilliam,
a remote upland town in the Western Cape. MacIver requested a move after only
four months: 'The climate is a healthy one [but] ... there are good reasons for my
wishing to leave the district ... income so small and expenses so great that ends
barely meet. Personal discomforts many and real and absolutely no compensatory
advantages.'[10] Although he was moved to another post, the transforming, indeed
life-giving, experience that McIver desperately needed from his new colonial
situation eluded him, and within three months he was dead, probably from
tuberculosis.

More fortunate was a young Irish colleague named Edward Garraway
(1865–1932). As a recently qualified Irish doctor, Garraway came in 1888 to
Millwood, a small mining community near Knysna in the Eastern Cape, to work
as an assistant district surgeon. He used an Irish network in the Cape to gain additional work as a medical assistant to a fellow countryman, Charles Gorman, in his
private general practice in Knysna. Soon after arriving in his new location, he
wrote a revealingly piece of self-description:

I was very young and I fear I looked it too, and I often felt rather sorry for these unfortunates ... who had to look to me for any assistance they might require in the event of illness or accident. ... Gorman bade me farewell, and started back [to Knysna] leaving a very homesick and thoroughly depressed 'GP' behind him.[11]

This young doctor's swift change to a colonial situation must have been characteristic of many youthful British medical migrants to southern Africa; he had not only to develop his identity and self-confidence as a medical practitioner, but also to adjust to a new environment. Initially he perceived this as 'a most forsaken spot': very hot, plagued by mosquitoes, and with a surgery invaded by scorpions and snakes.[12] However, he found compensating advantages in the colonial sporting life, organising his medical commitments to enable him to spend long hours shooting small game. Equally, like other Cape doctors practising in remote rural areas, he learned to be self-reliant and to develop a considerable range of clinical skills.

There were varied ways in which Cape doctors like Garraway became 'agents of empire': district surgeons identified themselves as occupying a front line not only in a fight against disease, but also in the advance of imperial civilisation (Van Heyningen 1989). Garraway was unusual in the extent of the abundant personal testimony he left in the form of letters and diaries, so that it is possible to see him constructing a new individuality that was shaped by his colonial surroundings, first for two years at Millwood, and then in his second professional position as a district surgeon at Kuruman on the northern Cape frontier. Garraway exemplified a process described by Woodward whereby migration tends to produce contested identities, with a search for ethnic certainties in a new, pluralistic racial situation (Woodward 1977: 16). He soon imbibed the pervasive racism of Cape society and asserted that 'one very soon loses one's exalted idea about the "poor negro" out here and see that the kinder you are to them the less they care about you'.[13] At Millwood he described Africans as 'the brutes', while at the old mission centre of Kuruman, he took a perverse pride in using 'nigger', a term imported from home, for the African, deliberately not adopting what he referred to as 'the missionary terminology of native'.[14] In this colonial discourse one might interpret him as attempting both to reassert his home identity and to highlight a gap he perceived between the superior white colonialist and the inferior black colonial subject.

In 1895 Garraway served as a civil surgeon in the notorious, imperialist adventure into the Afrikaner Republics, led by another British emigrant doctor, Leander Starr Jameson (1853–1917), and thus known as the Jameson Raid.[15] Garraway recorded of his involvement: 'January 2, 1896. The most awful night I hope ever to put in.'[16] Such military service was characteristic of many South African doctors. A contemporary medical immigrant from England, William Darley Hartley (1854–1934), went to the Cape in 1878 and, as a fervent imperialist, managed to serve in no fewer than six wars.[17] This kind of frequent military service led to a pronounced surgical proficiency, resulting in good all-round ability in surgery and medicine within the profession.

It also produced two other important elements in professional identities: flexibility and a resilient capacity to survive difficulties. Like Garraway and many of his colleagues, Darley Hartley was a peripatetic doctor. He was forced out of his first practice location in East London near the eastern frontier, as drought conditions meant his patients could not pay their bills. He then spent four years in a salaried appointment as district surgeon at Cathcart, before moving back to East London, where he stayed for a decade, then relocated to Cape Town. Darley Hartley became Editor of the *South African Medical Journal* (1884–9) and Founder-Editor of the *South African Medical Record* (1903–26), where he ran the periodical side by side with a medical agency advertising appointments and practices. He managed to make this sufficiently successful to give up medical practice for full-time journalism and medical politics. To an unusual extent there was an almost complete elision between his personal and professional personas. He was dedicated wholeheartedly to the advancement of collective medical interests, and his weekly editorials became the voice of the colonial profession through his advocacy of solidarity with British interests, skilful medical entrepreneurialism, and high standards of medical ethics. Darley Hartley became the doyen of the profession and on his retirement was awarded the first Gold Medal of the Medical Association of South Africa. He died a few years later in South Africa.

Whether émigrés retired to the 'home country' or stayed in South Africa was very much a matter of individual preference, and in any case numbers returning to the United Kingdom were small. Garraway, like Darley Hartley, ended up on the inside track of colonial appointments, as Resident Commissioner first of Bechuanaland, and then of Basutoland, for which he was knighted. Retiring to Ireland, Garraway might have reflected on how four decades of service in southern Africa had elevated him from being the obscure son of a respectable yet penurious military family into one of the county elite.

The cases of doctors who moved to South Africa have been used to discuss the issue of transformed identities created by migration from metropole to colony. What of movement in the opposite direction? Shorter-period migration to the UK was more common because many doctors who had been born in South Africa came to do their initial or postgraduate training in Britain, particularly before home-based medical training for whites became available in the 1920s. One such individual was Johann Balthazar Knobel (1853–1931), who chose to train at the University of Glasgow, where he qualified in 1877 and later completed an MD thesis in 1902. Born into an Afrikaner mercantile family in the Cape Colony, Knobel soon went to practice in the Afrikaner Republics of the Orange Free State and the Transvaal, where he also became a personal medical attendant of President Kruger of the Transvaal Republic.

In the South African War of 1899 to 1902 Knobel's political loyalties were with the Afrikaners, and so he fought against the British. But his professional identity had been profoundly shaped by his British medical training. In his self-presentation of his work as a general practitioner in Pretoria, analysed in his MD thesis, Knobel emphasised that his mental benchmark in evaluating a case was his earlier training. In discussing a case he would write that 'the most noticeable divergence from the normal routine as taught me at Glasgow University is' before going on to discuss a case's unusual features (Knobel 1902: 9). Knobel's multiple allegiances appear to have informed a professional detachment that was useful in dealing with the culturally diverse customs of his patients who included Dutch and German Afrikaners, as well as English, Jewish and African patients. He seems to have been even-handedly critical about his patients' preferred practices in the sickroom or predilections for types of medicine, whether he was castigating the over-crowded sickroom preferred by Afrikaner households or disparaging harmful ingredients in indigenous medicines used by Africans (Knobel 1902: 16, 24).

Non-whites were denied a medical training within South Africa until the 1940s. But small numbers managed to train in Britain and elsewhere, and their experiences provided another mapping of how race related to identity. They revealed ways in which the racism practised by Garraway and his colleagues might subdue or constrain the self in South Africa, but showed that the hitherto marginal colonial subject could be revitalised by a different environment. An Indian doctor stated that his time during training in Scotland had been 'a breath of fresh air. There is no question of a colour bar. It was a democratic society – we were free to move about without being kicked or humiliated' (Hey 1961: 28). Later, when a South African training for black doctors was provided, and in the context of the Black Consciousness Movement developing among the unprecedented concentration of intelligent young blacks on the campus, an African woman, Mamphele Ramphele, commented of Natal Medical School that it 'offered an environment for the transformation of my life ... I began to understand and interpret my own personal experiences of racism and oppression ... till then I had not fully grasped the relation between the personal and the political' (Ramphele 1995: 57). Here the training environment presented opportunities for the realisation and affirmation of black identity. Ironically, some white South African doctors had argued earlier that foreign training of blacks would deracialise them, so that they would wish to treat white patients and so become professional competitors in what was perceived to be an over-crowded medical market in South Africa (Digby 2006).

Medical practice in South Africa remained overwhelmingly private practice, so that there was not the reconstruction of identity experienced by British GPs following the development of insurance-based healthcare in 1911 and 1946–8 (discussed below.) This was despite the fact that during the Second World War both countries were discussing major health reforms, with each taking an interest in the reforming ideas of the other. After reading the visionary South African Gluckman Report of 1944, which advocated a thorough implementation of social medicine through the national development of health centres, one British official commented: 'This is a report that shows us what we should be doing!' (quoted in Marks 1997: 452). Although South Africa created a small number of health centres on the Gluckman model, most were short-lived. Gluckman's progressive vision of integrating doctors in community-based healthcare teams in order to improve the neglected health of the black population soon disintegrated within the ideologically hostile climate of the apartheid regime after 1948.

Forging local British medical identities

In 1884 the *Lancet* had warned that 'the [Medical] Register shows a steady increase in the number of persons registering annually ... an increase confirmed by the competition in the profession and the obvious excess of practitioners' (26 July 1884: 159). It was not only in new lands like South Africa that doctors had to extend their personal and professional attributes in order to survive. In Britain doctors had to expand professional boundaries by carving out new practices through appointments, and attempting to recruit new classes of patients by creating novel social identities.

We have seen that financial pressure was particularly acute during economically depressed years, like those in the 1880s and 1890s and again during the 1920s and 1930s. This led many to experiment with successive practice locations before finding a financially rewarding niche. Here doctors might adopt opportunistic strategies that drew on their own religious and ethnic backgrounds, political or military connections, or even sporting interests to develop social connections that resulted in paid appointments. These not only produced useful income but also gave a higher profile in the community. Amongst the most widely held appointments were those of medical officer to a poor law union, or part-time medical officer of health. Selection as a school medical officer offered another career option, as did an appointment as a police surgeon or a post office surgeon, whilst there were also industrial posts in factories, quarries, works, mines, and railway or canal companies (Digby 1999: 79–82).

Successful strategies of social networking with face-to-face contact in a range of activities led the doctor to integrate with community activities, so constructing a local public identity. The *Lancet* recorded what it perceived to be 'the steady growth of the influence of medical men in society' (16 March 1901: 797). To establish a reputation and to foster trust resulted in public identification with the community, both in the views of local people and the doctor's self-estimation. As a result a few exceptional GPs might have a hospital ward named after them, or have their memory perpetuated through a portrait hung in the local infirmary.[18] Heroic exertion was also recognised. The large illuminated address presented to Dr Reidy of Llanbadrach, by five hundred subscribers, was a nice example of the high regard of 'their' doctor held by a Welsh mining community. Surrounded by hand-painted pictures of the doctor attending injured men underground, it read 'Assiduous attention to the call of duty and your readiness and fitness at all times and hours to respond to that call have secured to you the lasting confidence and gratitude of the community'.[19]

The contribution that GPs made to their local societies through long service stimulated communities to recognise it formally by personal testimonials, material gifts such as a retirement present of a purse of sovereigns, or a handsome cheque.[20] And if fifty years of service or retirement signalled rites of passage in the doctor's relationship with the community, so too did a beloved doctor's funeral. 'We are here today lamenting the passing of "the Doctor," for as such he was known to all of us; he was a doctor *par excellence* who spent his life and himself without stint for those who he loved and willingly served' (*BMJ* I, 1940: 509–10). That communities turned out to pay their last respects attested to the doctor's role where s/he was identified as a central pillar of the community. Dr Bucknill, for example, was a member of a family of GPs who had served the English Midlands town of Rugby for over a century, and who himself acted as a GP for four decades. On his death over 2,000 people gathered for his funeral procession (BMJ II, 1881: 1002).

Private and public in Britain: the ambiguity of familial identities

In small British towns multi-generational medical practices of family dynasties were well-known (*BMJ* III, 1970: 351; II, 1920: 415; I, 1940: 154). Equally, British medical schools recruited the sons and daughters of earlier medical graduates. So it has become a commonplace to say that 'medicine ran in families'. But looking at the actual incidence of family-based practices at any given point in time indicates that before 1910 only one in eight practices (12 percent) were family practices, defined as having more than one family member. Historically, it was comparatively rare for localities to be able to generate enough income to support more than one doctor, so that even if a family practice was desired, it was not feasible. After 1910 family practices increased to one in seven (16 percent), probably in response to augmented income from the national health insurance scheme implemented in 1913. So only a small minority of general practitioners worked professionally within family partnership (Digby 1999: 77). The term 'family practice' is ambiguous, however, because of its multiple meanings: it can also mean that the doctor's practice aspired to treat whole families as their patients. There was an enduring contrast between the ideal of a family doctor embodying caring, sympathetic and friendly qualities towards patients, and the cold impersonality of scientific hospital medicine (Loudon 1984).

The term 'family doctor' is perhaps most accurately applied in a context that few have analysed directly, but one that shaped both personal and professional identity. For most British generalists before the advent of public grants for health centres in the mid-1960s, the doctor's private house doubled as professional premises. That general practice was a cottage industry was thus literally true in terms of bricks and mortar. This was one important factor that made it all too easy for a professional identity to submerge a private one, and the complex interface of public duty and private life was at its most visible in the doctor's house. This meant that the doctor's family necessarily shared in the dialectic between the public and private within the organisational life of the practice. From nights disturbed by the speaking tube connecting the front door to the bedroom, to days punctuated by patients' calls, the doctor's spouse and children were always conscious that the term 'family doctor' had an additional meaning. The 'doctor's wife' felt the asymmetric pull of her husband's occupation in functioning as an 'incorporated' wife, where – as Callan has noted – there was an interpenetration of institutional and conjugal structures and identities (Callan 1984).

Between the demise of the doctor's apprentice in the 1880s and the availability of government funding for auxiliary staff in the 1960s, the frequently unpaid, informal work of the spouse ensured the viability of the practice. Delivering valuable material services through acting as gatekeeper in answering the door or the telephone, providing 'spot' diagnoses of simpler medical conditions, or doubling as secretary, bookkeeper and office manager, and (if in possession of a professional qualification) also acting as nursing assistant or dispenser as well, the spouse was both marital partner and informal professional partner. The wife might also have an important cultural role in the public representation of the doctor, through making social calls and leaving visiting cards. In those rare cases where it was the wife and not the husband who was the doctor, the husband did not normally play a similarly supporting role.

The importance of social settings as frames of meaning for the relationship between self-image and public or professional image is well known (Jenkins 1996, esp. chap. 8 for a useful discussion). The frequent merging of the familial and the professional in the life of many British doctors was quite revealing, and an accompanying lack of interests outside the medical vocation (especially for the busy urban doctor) also suggested the person-defining power of medical occupation. Some general practitioners were like Dr Crawford, whose 'daily work [was] his sole hobby', or like Dr Joy, who did not take any holiday in 55 years of practice, because 'the pursuit of his profession furnished him with all the recreation he needed' (*BMJ* I, 1940: 509-10; II, 1880: 34). A minority had a more rounded lifestyle in which self-identity was not wholly collapsed into a professional one. Those with well-developed hobbies were in the group who welcomed retirement, as did Dr Court, who retired promptly on the morning of his sixtieth birthday so that he could pursue archaeology, fishing, and shooting (*BMJ* II, 1960: 1813). Country doctors working in lowland areas where the population, and hence patient distribution, was reasonably dense, often managed to combine their work and their interests: pursuing sporting pastimes or advancing knowledge of natural history during visits to the homes of their patients. They sustained a higher leisure preference than was possible in the busier lives of urban doctors, centred on a high throughput of patients and frequently held surgeries.

But country doctors working in upland areas, and thus with widely scattered patients, spent so much time travelling to visit them that they had few opportunities for leisure interests. Thus, like urban doctors, they tended to put all their energies into their professional vocation. These doctors might fear retirement and the need to invest life with more than professional work. Revealingly a female GP, Dr Bensusan-Butt of Colchester, commented that 'I would rather wear out, than rust out'.[21] But this driven professional lifestyle had its personal costs. A substantial proportion of doctors, varying from two- to three-fifths, dropped down dead in the course of their work. In this they fulfilled their desired destiny, since obituaries frequently recorded that a general practitioner 'died, as he wished, in full harness' (for example, *BMJ* I, 1920: 421)

Reconstructed identities: the impact of the British state

During the twentieth century identities of GPs were shaped increasingly by more impersonal institutional factors. In 1911 a national system of health insurance (NHI) provided revenue tied to low-earning (largely adult male) patients for GPs who signed up as its 'panel' doctors. In financial importance this grew to be more significant than revenue from appointments based in specific communities. As a result, local factors became less important in the construction of professional identities, so that there were diminishing numbers of generalists who practised in the same region as they had been born and trained. Instead, the secure capitation payments for their panel of working-class patients enabled entrants to the profession to set up a practice anywhere in the country (Digby Forthcoming 2006b).

Twentieth-century GPs were thus much less likely than their Victorian predecessors to pursue their careers on the basis of local and regional connection, or of personal networks. Obtaining income from national bodies also had other implications, notably the growing importance of a gatekeeping role by doctors. However, when it was necessary to testify to the fitness or otherwise of their patients' eligibility for insurance-related benefits, conflicts of interest might reshape the simple loyalties of the traditional patient-doctor relationship. Equally, the NHI doctor ceased to be a freestanding medic possessing a distinctive social identity once the necessity for bureaucratic returns, as well as periodic official inspection of records and practices, impinged on independence. And the kind of fast throughput, involving assembly-line methods, found necessary for managing large numbers of panel patients, may well have falsified idealistic expectations of practice fostered earlier by medical schools, so reshaping professional self-image (Digby 1999: 252–3, 313–22).

Ultimately about three-quarters of the profession became panel doctors, although most had mixed practices including both panel and private patients. NHI income provided a stable basis of revenue that ensured economic survival for almost all, and relative prosperity for many. This contrasted with the situation in the decades preceding the 1911 act when an unregulated output by medical schools had resulted in a proleterianised group of 'sixpenny' and 'shilling' doctors, who extended the medical market by charging low fees to working-class patients. Their substandard premises in converted shops, failure to examine patients, and predilection for prescribing stock bottles of medicine, were held by their colleagues to have subverted traditional standards, thus compromising professional identity (Digby 1994: 168–9). In contrast, the inter-war era of mixed panel and private practice created the markers of a middle-class, prosperous social identity for many generalists. Lifestyle images included possession of a substantial house, one or two cars in the garage, children sent to private school, a maidservant to open the front door to middle-class patients, and an afternoon on the golf course once a week. In altering the trajectories and processes on which many GPs had customarily organised their professional identities, the effects of the NHI scheme were pervasive (Digby and Bosanquet 1989).

Larger structural factors also influenced further changes in GPs' identities after the National Health Service of 1946–8 brought many more patients – women, children, and middle-class men – into a service free at the point of access. The effect on self-identity of a commercialisation of relationships has been noted by Craib (1998). The unison with which GPs celebrated the free service for their patients in 1948, when money no longer came between patients and doctors, suggests the historical strain that this had once imposed on professional aspiration and identity (Craib 1998: 3). Anxieties by doctors that they would become dependent civil servants under the new organisation were not realised, although some resented a growth in workload resulting from new groups of patients accessing medical care, as well as an increased burden of bureaucratic paperwork. In drawing unfavourable comparisons with the lucrative NHS contracts won by specialists and consultants, initial poor self-esteem and low morale made GPs think of themselves as the Cinderellas of the NHS (Digby 1999: chap. 13).

Key changes in general practice were concentrated less on the introduction of the NHS in 1948 than was the case with other sectors of the health service. Thus it is relevant to discuss related changes which took place in the following two decades. These involved a significant shift in GPs' own perceptions and realisation of their identities. During the 1950s and 1960s key organisational changes occurred, including: the adoption of appointment systems and the holding of fewer surgeries, which relieved the unremitting flow of patients; a mid-century growth in partnerships which enabled a sharing of night and weekend duties; a growth in government-assisted, purpose-built premises (from the mid-1960s), thus enabling the physical separation of home from work; and an increase in ancillary support staff (again assisted by government grants), which freed the doctor's spouse from a 24 hour per day commitment to the practice. All contributed to the development of a new, private space and a private identity. In turn this produced a more negative attitude by younger colleagues toward the lifestyles and identities of their predecessors before 1948, because the latter had seen their work as an all-consuming goal. Obituaries thus spoke disapprovingly of them belonging to the 'old school', who were 'completely absorbed' in work or who had 'unlimited hours of work, [and] instant availability' (*BMJ* I, 1960: 1817; *BMJ* II, 1970: 487).

Conclusion

A variety of perspectives have been utilised to examine overlapping dimensions and evolutionary changes in generalists' identities. The situational character of collective identity, and the historical specificities of individual identity, indicate some of the reasons which facilitated the fluid and negotiable character of GPs' social identities (Jenkins 1996: 102). Whereas in nineteenth-century Britain the general practitioner made considerable effort to construct a distinctive social image that would appeal to a local community, collective health insurance in the twentieth century undercut this rationale. The heroic individualism of the Victorian doctors portrayed so dramatically in the paintings by Hardy and Fildes therefore contrasts with the more anonymous doctors of the twentieth century, whose distinctive aspirations were constrained by the standardising impact of bureaucratic NHI or NHS regulations. So larger structural factors – whether of state health schemes or of colonialism – impacted on collective identity. In South Africa professional identities were shaped by relationships to empire, and were also heavily conditioned by non-medical factors, notably endemic racism. Unlike British generalists, those in South Africa had greater financial independence from the state, because of the failure of the Gluckman projected reforms of 1944, which would have given a system of improved patient accessibility (particularly for black patients) not dissimilar to the inclusive aims of the NHS in Britain. This financial situation meant that general practice medicine in South Africa continued as private practice; thus, self-reliant entrepreneurism continued to be a defining feature of the identity of any South African GP, in a way that was no longer the case for a British GP under the NHS.

Notes

The author appreciates the financial support given to this research by the Wellcome Trust and by Oxford Brookes University, and the helpful comments made by the Editor, by members of the seminar on medical identities held in the University of Oxford, and by the late Charles Feinstein.

1. Obituary for Dr B.M. Lewis, qualified 1888, who practised at Pontypridd, Glamorgan for nearly fifty years.
2. D. Huskie, MA, MB. FRCP Ed., died 1943.
3. See, for example, the historical depiction of country doctors in North Wales in Morris Jones 1961.
4. See Hall, 1990 for a more detailed discussion of the process of identification and reconstitution.
5. For a general discussion of this topic see Goffman 1971; Jenkins 1996, chap. 13.
6. Obituary, *Medical Women's Federation Quarterly Newsletter*, 23 March 1923. O'Connor practised in Stratford, East London.
7. Wellcome Library Archives, London, GP 29/2/6 for Margaret Norton (MB, ChB, Birmingham, 1939).
8. University of Cape Town Archives, BC 700, letter to Dr Stewart 21 August 1898. Waterston had been a medical missionary before becoming a GP.
9. CA, NA/471, African Affairs Department applications and letters from district surgeons (1879–97), letters from Dr MacIver, 14 May and 22 July 1895.
10. CA, NA/471, letter from Dr MacIver to Rose Innes, 10 June 1896.

11. Rhodes House, Oxford, Garraway papers, MSS Afr.s.1610, vol. 12, folios 188–91. For a fuller account of Garraway's career see Digby 2006a, chaps 2 and 6.
12. MSS Afr.s.1610, vol. 1, ff. 12 and 24, letters 21 March and 30 March 1888.
13. MSS Afr.s.1610, vol. 1, f. 81, letter of 6 July 1888; vol. 2, f. 121, letter of 1 May 1890.
14. MSS Afr.s.1610, vol. 1, ff. 52 and 54, letter of 2 June 1888; vol. 3, f. 43, letter of 9 March 1891.
15. Jameson was a close associate of Cecil Rhodes, and his economic and political activities (including Premiership of the Cape Colony from 1904 to 1908) gradually superseded his medical ones.
16. Diary extracts were published in *Harper's New Monthly Magazine*, November 1896, p. 818.
17. For a fuller account of Darley Hartley's career see Digby 1994.
18. Nottinghamshire Record Office, DD 1440/26/3, scrapbook on Dr Ringrose; Williams, 1979: 7; *BMJ*, I, 1930: 671; II, 1950: 1063–4.
19. Mid-Glamorgan Record Office, D/D X 543/1, illuminated address to William Augustus Reidy, 1902.
20. *BMJ* II, 1890: 1335–6; II, 1890: 251–2; I, 1910: 607, 1089–90; II, 1930: 983; I, 1960: 353.
21. Greater Manchester Record Office, Medical Women's Federation Scrapbook for Dr Ben-susan-Butt, who was a GP from 1907 to 1950.

References

Archival sources

Cape Archives, NA/471, African Affairs Department applications and correspondence concerning district surgeons (1879–97).
Greater Manchester Record Office, Medical Women's Federation Scrapbook.
Mid-Glamorgan Record Office, D/D X 543/1, illuminated address to William Augustus Reidy, 1902.
Nottinghamshire Record Office, DD 1440/26/3, scrapbook on Dr Ringrose.
Rhodes House, Oxford, MSS Afr.s.1610, Garraway papers.
University of Cape Town Archives, BC 700, correspondence of J. Waterston.
Wellcome Library Archives, London, GP 29/2/6, Margaret Norton transcript.

Printed sources

1908. *BMA Presidential Addresses, 1888–1908.* Cape Town.
Anderson, B. 1983. *Imagined Communities: Reflections on the Origins and Spread of Nationalism.* London: Verso.
British Medical Journal (BMH).
Bewell, A. 1999. *Romanticism and Colonial Disease.* Baltimore and London: Johns Hopkins University Press.
Callan, H. 1984. 'Introduction'. In *The Incorporated Wife.* H. Callan and S. Ardener (eds). London: Croom Helm.
Castells, M. 1997. *The Power of Identity.* Oxford: Blackwell.
Craib, I. 1998. *Experiencing Identity.* London: Sage.
Digby, A. and N. Bosanquet. 1989. 'Doctors and Patients in an Era of National Health Insurance and Private Practice'. *Economic History Review*, 2nd series, XLI 74–94.

Digby, A. 1994. *Making a Medical Living: Doctors and Patients in the English Market for Medicine, 1720–1911.* Cambridge: Cambridge University Press.

——— 1995. '"A Medical El Dorado"? Colonial Medical Incomes and Practice at the Cape'. *Social History of Medicine,* VIII 463–79.

——— 1999. *The Evolution of British General Practice, 1850–1948.* Oxford: Oxford University Press.

——— 2004. 'Making a Medical Living: The Economics of Medical Practice in the Cape, circa 1860–1910'. In *A Social History of the Nineteenth Century Cape Doctor.* H.J. Deacon, H. Phillips and E. Van Heyningen (eds). Amsterdam: Rodopi 249–79.

——— 2005. 'Early Black Doctors in South Africa'. *Journal of African History* 46.

——— 2006a. *Diversity and Division in Medicine: Health Care in South Africa from the 1800s.* Oxford: Peter Lang.

——— 2006b. 'The Economic and Medical Significance of the British National Health Insurance Act, 1911'. In *Financing British Medicine, 1750–2000.* S. Sheard and M. Gorsky (eds). London: Routledge, Studies in the Social History of Medicine.

Eliot, G. 1996. *Middlemarch: A Study of Provincial Life.* Oxford: World's Classics edition. Oxford: Oxford University Press.

Fildes, V. 1968. *Luke Fildes, RA: A Victorian Painter.* London: Michael Joseph.

Goffman, E. 1971. *The Presentation of Self in Everyday Life.* Harmondsworth: Penguin.

——— 1974. *Frame Analysis.* New York: Harper and Row.

Good, B.T. 1994. *Medicine, Rationality and Experience: An Anthropological Perspective.* Cambridge: Cambridge University Press.

Hall, S. 1990. 'Cultural Identity and Diaspora'. *In Identity, Community, Culture, Difference.* J. Rutherford (ed.). London: Lawrence and Wishart 222–37.

Hey, P.D. 1961. *The Rise of the Natal Indian Elite.* Pietermaritzburg: Natal Witness.

Huskie, D. 1938. 'Impressions and Experiences of a Country Doctor in the 'Nineties and After'. *Transactions of the Medico-Chirurgical Society of Edinburgh* 10–12.

Jalland, P. (ed.). 1989. *Octavia Wilberforce: The Autobiography of a Pioneer Woman Doctor.* London: Cassell.

Jenkins, R. 1996. *Social Identity.* London: Routledge.

Johnson, T.J. and M. Caygill. 1972–3. 'The British Medical Association and its Overseas Branches: A Short History'. *Journal of Imperial and Commonwealth History* I 303–29.

Loudon, I. 1984. 'The Concept of the Family Doctor'. *Bulletin of the History of Medicine* 58 347–62.

Malleson, H. 1919. *A Woman Doctor: Mary Murdoch of Hull.* London: Sidgwick and Jackson.

Medical Women's Federation Quarterly Newsletter.

Marks, S. 1997. 'South Africa's Early Experiment in Social Medicine: Its Pioneers and Policies'. *American Journal of Public Health* 87 453–9.

Morris Jones, H. 1961. 'The Country Doctors of Fifty Years Ago'. *Country Quest,* Autumn issue 21–2.

Oosthuizen, S.F. 1957. 'The Numbers and Distribution of Medical Practitioners in the Union'. *South African Medical Journal* (23 March): 289–91.

Phillips, H. 2004. 'Home Taught from Abroad: The Training of the Cape Doctor'. In *A Social History of the Nineteenth Century Cape Doctor.* H. Deacon, H. Phillips and E. Van Heyningen (eds). Amsterdam: Rodopi.

Ramphele, M. 1995. *Across Boundaries: The Journey of a South African Woman Leader.* New York: Feminist Press.

Rosen, G. 1967. 'People, Disease and Emotion: Some Newer Problems for Research in Medical History'. *Bulletin of the History of Medicine* 4: 5–23.

Rutherford, J. 1990a. 'A Place Called Home: Identity and the Cultural Politics of Difference'. In *Identity, Community, Culture, Difference*. J. Rutherford (ed.). London: Lawrence and Wishart.

———— (ed.). 1990b. *Identity, Community, Culture, Difference*. London: Lawrence and Wishart.

St John, C. 1935. *Christine Murrell, MD: Her Life and Work*. London: Williams and Norgate.

South African Medical Journal (SAMJ).

Trollope, A. 1980. *Dr Thorne*. Oxford: Oxford University Press, World's Classics Edition.

Union of South Africa Parliamentary Papers. UG 32 1912. *Census 1911, Part V Occupations*.

Van Heyningen, E. 1989. 'Agents of Empire: The Medical Profession in the Cape Colony, 1880–1910'. *Medical History*, 33 450–71.

Walker, E. 2001. '"Conservative Pioneers": The Formation of the South Africa Society of Medical Women'. *Social History of Medicine*, 14 483–505.

Wallen, M. 2004. *City of Health, Fields of Disease: Revolution in the Poetry, Medicine and Philosophy of Romanticism*. Aldershot: Ashgate

Webster, C. 1988. *The Health Services since the War. Vol. 1. Problems of Health Care. The National Health Service before 1957*. London: H.M.S.O.

Williams, J.H. 1979. *GPs of Barry, 1885–1979*. Barry: Barry Medical Society.

Wood, C. 1988. *Paradise Lost: Paintings of English Country Life and Landscape, 1850–1914*. London: Barrie and Jenkins.

Woodward, K. In *Identity and Difference*. K. Woodyand (ed.). 1997. '*Concepts of Identity and Difference*'. London: Open University and Sage.

Unpublished sources

Knobel, J.B. 1902. 'Some Remarks on the Professional Experiences of a General Medical Practitioner in Pretoria, Transvaal'. MD thesis, University of Glasgow.

2

PHARMACISTS AND OTHER DRUG-PROVIDERS IN CAMBODIA: IDENTITIES AND EXPERIENCES

Ing-Britt Trankell and Jan Ovesen

Introduction

Like many developing countries in the last decades, Cambodia has seen a dramatic increase in the availability of biomedical pharmaceuticals. It is a commonplace observation that, globally, the production and marketing of pharmaceuticals is very big business indeed, and that it is only tenuously linked to the real healthcare needs of the ordinary population in developing countries. National as well as global economic and political inequalities are directly reflected in the standard and availability of healthcare, including people's access to adequate and sufficient medicines. Situations in which poor people in poor countries are deprived of proper healthcare and medication have been documented by Paul Farmer (2003) in terms of structural violence; likewise, Nguyen and Peschard (2003: 448–9) have characterised the health impact of transnational inequalities as the production of a 'striking culture of indifference to affliction in areas of extreme inequality' where 'the poor trade in their long-term health for survival while the rich … are able to purchase better health'.

In this chapter we focus on the resources that ordinary Cambodians – poor people in a poor country – have for meeting their immediate medical needs. We offer an ethnography of the distribution and consumption of medicines and look at how biomedical pharmaceuticals and their purveyors interact with indigenous remedies and their providers. When seeking cure for minor ailments or relief from anxieties, the majority of the Cambodian population, both urban and rural, will go to a nearby pharmacy, to a local drugseller, or an indigenous healer. Even for more serious conditions, relief is often first sought at a pharmacy, rather than from a physician.[1]

The apparently massive dominance of modern pharmaceuticals on the Cambodian drug market does not imply that the consumers and providers of these pharmaceuticals are necessarily 'modern' people, any more than clients of 'traditional' healers are completely pre-modern. Nguyen and Peschard have proposed a distinction between the premodern, modern and a-modern medical worlds. Characteristic of medical premodernity is the absence of an institutional distinction between therapeutic and socio-political space, between illness and sorcery, healing and exorcism. Medical modernity implies 'political spaces of health, where misfortune is managed through specialized therapeutic institutions' (Nguyen and Peschard 2003: 448); while in the a-modern condition, 'the lines between political and therapeutic power are once again blurred' (op. cit.). We suggest that the notion of a-modernity well describes the medical situation in contemporary Cambodia. Apart from the 'blurred lines' – which stem from and reflect global and national political-economic and medical inequalities – the a-modern Cambodian medical world is characterised by syntheses of premodern and modern elements.

The majority of the Cambodian population still orient themselves in light of a premodern medical world, in which physical or mental illness is associated with social or moral transgression; healing is a process actively engaged in by both healer and sufferer, and leads to the mending of social and spiritual relationships, thus restoring the health of the person. Even among educated urbanites who may express disdain for 'traditional' medical practices, a modern medical world-view informed exclusively by the principles of biomedicine cannot be taken for granted. Indigenous healers are referred to as *kru* ('teacher', from the Sanskrit *guru*), and the element of teaching is central in the therapeutic process, in which the sick person is expected to be 'taught' how to get well in the course of a diagnostic dialogue. The modality of this dialogue is spiritual, but its therapeutic import is social, psychological and psychosomatic. The dialogue is negotiated in the sense that decisions about the diagnosis, and the course of therapy, must be based on a consensus between the *kru*, the patient and his or her relatives, and the spirits.

In the Cambodian cultural conception, the healing process consists of three phases: finding the cause of the illness through negotiating the diagnostic dialogue (diagnosis); prescribing the proper medical (herbal and spiritual) treatment (cure); and feedback by socially expressing the conclusion of the process (acknowledgment). The first two elements are, of course, equally prominent in biomedical practice, even if the patient's role is less active in the processes, and the social, moral and spiritual dimensions are generally neglected. The element of acknowledgement, on the other hand, is usually missing altogether from biomedical practice, which may be one reason why many patients experience a marked sense of unfulfilment even after a 'successful' biomedical cure. Given that the indigenous conception of the healing process can be seen to follow the pattern of a classic rite of passage, the sense of unfulfilment is understandable when the final phase of social reincorporation has not been performed. An acknowledgement may range from a modest token of respect to the healer, through an offering ceremony at the temple, to an elaborate sacrificial ritual with the participation of numerous spirit mediums (cf. Trankell 2003). In the modern biomedical world, on the other hand, a fixed payment is required in advance, and occasional gifts from patients to doctors after treatment are not necessarily received in the same spirit as they are given. Most people therefore make their acknowledgement as offerings to the temple rather than to the doctor. But even official representatives of biomedical modernity may make allowance for the premodern orientation of their patients; at the provincial hospital in Kampong Chhnang, for example, there is a spirit shrine in the reception area where patients can make small offerings, and the large bo-tree in the courtyard is always endowed with incense sticks, bearing witness to the synthesis of modern and premodern aspects of medical care.

Historical background

The products and marketing efforts of the transnational pharmaceutical industry have reached consumers only fairly recently in Cambodia, given its economic marginality.[2] Yet, the availability of biomedical pharmaceuticals is not a recent phenomenon. Cambodians were first introduced to Western medicine during the French colonial period (1863–1953). As part of their colonial 'civilising mission', the French made quite serious efforts in the field of public health (Trankell and Ovesen 2004). The colonial medical service was expressly aimed primarily at the healthcare of the 'natives', and at least up until the 1920s, the promotion of European medicine and pharmaceuticals was high on the agenda of the colonial government.

During the latter part of the colonial period and well into independence, increasing numbers of Cambodian medical and pharmaceutical (as well as other) students were sent for studies in France. During the Prince Sihanouk regime (1955–70), medical and pharmaceutical education within the country was a significant element in the modernisation programme, and a large number of hospitals, dispensaries and health-centres were opened throughout the country (Desbarats 1995: 153–5). Medical treatment was officially free of charge, but during the country's economic decline from the mid-1960s, corruption among government officials and chief physicians undermined this policy (Martin 1994: 70–1). This tendency was exacerbated during the civil war under the Lon Nol regime (1970–5) and matters were made even worse by decreasing imports of pharmaceuticals; what little was available was very expensive (Brun 1998: 23), and only those who could afford an inflated bill would receive treatment. For most people the medical situation had become similar to the precolonial one when it was left to indigenous healers, spirit mediums and Buddhist monks to take care of people's health.

The Khmer Rouge regime (1975–9, a period colloquially referred to as 'Pol Pot') entailed a further deterioration of the medical and pharmaceutical situation. As soon as Khmer Rouge forces had captured Phnom Penh and other major cities (in April 1975), the urban population, consisting mainly of traders, civil servants and intellectuals, was ordered to leave for the countryside in order to participate in the revolution through forced agricultural labour. Even patients in the hospitals were evicted and many died in the process (Martin 1994: 171–2). It is estimated that during the four years of the Pol Pot regime, 80 percent of those evacuees were killed or died from malnutrition and/or exhaustion. Intellectuals were treated especially harshly because of the revolutionaries' ideological stance, that equated them with 'class enemies', and their general disdain for 'bourgeois' education. A large number of educated people, among them many physicians and pharmacists, were killed (De Nike et al. 2000: 326–7); many others perished while serving as slave-labourers.

It is commonly believed that modern medical services were completely abolished during Pol Pot, and that with few exceptions, hospitals were abandoned; thus David Chandler, prominent historian of Cambodia, states that Khmer Rouge practices included 'a rejection of Western-style medicine' (1993: 259), and that 'tens of thousands of Cambodians died … owing to the regime's refusal to import medicine' (op. cit. p.249). This is inaccurate, however. First, while it is certainly true that a large number of people died from inadequate medical care, our interviews with former Khmer Rouge medical personnel have established that existing major hospitals were used by the Pol Pot regime, and documents in the Cambodian National Archives show that pharmaceuticals were imported in substantial quantities. But the major hospitals and the imported pharmaceuticals were not for everyone. As Chandler has noted, hierarchy was by no means abolished by the revolution, 'but high positions were held by different categories of people than before and were no longer expressed in terms of money, possessions, or prerevolutionary titles. Instead, those with power and status … had access to [the] commodities that most of the population lacked: food, weapons and information' (op. cit. p.241). We only need to add medicine to the list of commodities to get the proper picture. Imported pharmaceuticals were stored in warehouses in Phnom Penh and Sihanoukville, from where they were distributed to the major hospitals, primarily in Phnom Penh and Battambang; these hospitals were reserved for the highest Khmer Rouge leadership and the treatment of complicated cases among revolutionary cadres.[3] Domestic pharmaceuticals (production of which had begun during the 1960s), now of increasingly inferior quality (because of the lack of qualified pharmacists), were dispensed to revolutionary cadres and other trusted individuals, while the remedy available to the great majority was herbal medicine manufactured as tablets, colloquially known as 'rabbit shit' (*ak tonsay*) as that was what they most resembled.[4] Second, the deterioration of the healthcare situation for the population at large was not related to any departure from modernity. On the contrary, the Pol Pot regime was in many ways decidedly 'modern' (cf. Marston 2002), and it provides a clear illustration of the fact that modernity does not necessarily entail progress or improvement. Khmer Rouge medical modernity defined illness bureaucratically as the inability to work, and a sick person was to be transferred from his/her ordinary working and social environment to a designated 'therapeutic' space, an infirmary (*munti pet*, 'medical office'). Formerly, illness had been very much a social concern, and care of the sick person was the prerogative primarily of his or her immediate family; only in serious cases was a sick person taken to hospital. The Khmer Rouge 'modernisation' of healthcare therefore required the establishment of a number of local infirmaries throughout the countryside; Buddhist temples, for example, were frequently converted into infirmaries.

When Vietnam invaded Cambodia in 1979 and installed a puppet regime, the People's Republic of Kampuchea (PRK), to replace the Khmer Rouge, restoration of the medical infrastructure was high on the list of government priorities. Surviving medical personnel were enrolled in refresher and/or crash courses in the provinces, and new students were admitted in significant numbers to the reopened medical faculty at the university in Phnom Penh. Physicians from Cuba, the GDR, Hungary, Poland and the USSR were also sent to assist their Vietnamese colleagues as advisers. In 1981, 'a total of 956 tonnes of medical equipment had been received from fraternal socialist countries and from humanitarian aid organizations' (Slocomb 2003: 173). However, the downside of such fraternal and humanitarian gestures was that the donors often used them as a way to get rid of their domestic surplus. As a current medical inspector at the Ministry of Health explained, the supplies came in 'boxes', and because of the urgent need and the lack of qualified personnel, the boxes were sent directly to the provinces without being inventoried or subjected to quality control.

Although, officially, there was no private healthcare sector during the PRK (1979–89), a fair number of boxes (from donations or from stockpiles in former Khmer Rouge warehouses) found their way to the private market, either sold for gold and jewellery[5] by Vietnamese army or civilian personnel, or simply by 'falling off a truck'. Rice and pharmaceuticals were the most precious commodities in the first years after the Vietnamese invasion; together with gold, they formed a triangular trade, carried out by Chinese and Sino-Khmer traders, as well as by Khmers. Many of the pharmacies that exist today were founded in the early 1980s on this sort of trade, conducted in the marketplaces from boxes or vegetable baskets.

At the same time, the state encouraged the development of indigenous herbal medicine as part of its nationalist ideology of self-sufficiency, which also had been on the agenda of the Khmer Rouge. Presumably inspired by the Chinese state-institutionalisation of 'traditional' medicine (Hsu 1999: 6–8), the government conscripted people who had served as herbalists during Pol Pot and put them to work at provincial and district hospitals or clinics, all of which were to have a medicinal garden attached to them. In that way, the state institutionalised the 'traditional' medical sector and integrated it into its modern medical worldview. The PRK, like the Pol Pot regime, thus evinced a non-capitalist medical modernity, in which the state kept the political control of a clearly demarcated therapeutic space, upheld its monopoly on violence, and reproduced, albeit less flagrantly, social and medical inequalities (see for example Martin 1994: 220–2).

With the Vietnamese withdrawal and the liberalisation of the economy in 1989, the 'grand narrative' of socialism finally lost its credibility, and with it went the visions of a great future for indigenous herbal medicine. Licensing of private pharmacies was introduced in 1988. After the general opening up of the country following the intervention of UNTAC (United Nations Transitional Authority in Cambodia) at the beginning of the 1990s, the US dollar became *de facto* the national currency. Pharmaceutical imports soared, and since the late 1990s about a dozen domestic pharmaceutical companies (engaged in production, as well as import and even export) are also active on the market.

With the intervention of UNTAC the country was thoroughly affected by globalisation, not only in economic terms of global capitalist market forces, but also in cultural terms. The massive influx of foreigners – UNTAC personnel amounted to more than 20,000 persons from all continents – brought with it bewildering cosmopolitan lifestyles and all sorts of consumer goods that contrasted sharply with the austere Vietnamese version of socialism that had reigned for more than a decade. To many people it appeared that by being exposed to this influx, their world had become literally fantastic, re-enchanted, but also more dangerous. As one of our informants put it, 'UNTAC released all the spirits'. We suggest that the arrival of global capitalist modernity paradoxically acted as a catalyst in the creation of an a-modern world. In the Cambodian medical world today, the lines between political and therapeutic power are certainly blurred: the Ministry of Health, like all other ministries, is severely limited in terms of human and financial resources, and international organisations and NGOs often compete with the government over therapeutic control. As for pharmaceutical control, it seems that all these parties often lose out to the pharmaceutical companies, whose commercial interests rarely coincide with those of either government or aid organisations.

The pharmaceutical infrastructure

Most village shops have a small selection of pharmaceuticals: amidst the dried noodles, biscuits, batteries, washing powder and candy, one will find jars of pills (painkillers, vitamins) and colourful capsules (supposedly antibiotics). When people in the village where we lived and worked needed remedies for minor ailments or a slight fever, they went to a shop in the small village market and bought a couple of pills or capsules, depending on what they could afford. For more serious illnesses, typically malaria or diarrhoea in children, they would call on our friend, Doctor Pham, the local 'injection doctor' (*pet phum*, 'village medic'), who offers treatment for 500 Riels (about US ¢15), plus the cost of medicine from his own small stock of pharmaceuticals. If his stock were depleted, he would write a 'prescription', i.e. a shopping list, to be filled by a pharmacy or drug shop in the district town 5 km away.

At all district centres there are several drug shops around the market. They all display the word 'pharmacy' and the associated sign, a green cross on a white background. But one should not expect to find a trained pharmacist behind the counter: officially, a pharmacy should have a license held by a professional pharmacist, but such people are few and far between in the countryside. Realising the need among the local population for access to pharmaceuticals – as well as the economic potential of the drug trade – district officials will not make unreasonable demands when mutually beneficial arrangements can be made. In actual fact, the majority of both pharmacies and drug shops are unlicensed. Thus, in the province of Kampong Chhnang, for example, there are 90 pharmacies and drug shops, of which only ten are licensed (seven pharmacies and three drug shops); nine of these, moreover, are located in the provincial capital.[6]

A small drug shop in our field area is run by a Khmer couple in their mid-forties; neither has any pharmacological education. For their small shop, the owners do not buy supplies from the various pharmaceutical companies whose vans pass

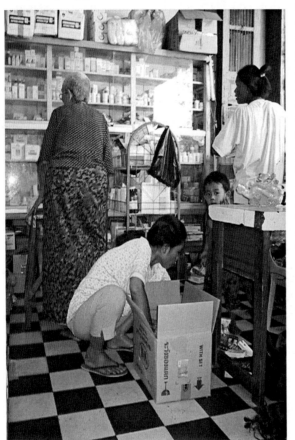

regularly: the companies only sell fairly large quantities, and the couple has little money and a modest sales volume. Instead, they get their supplies from the man's elder sister who is a trained pharmacist working at the provincial health centre; she also runs her own private pharmacy in the provincial capital. The sister may offer short-term credit, unlike the companies, and she also recommends what to buy for the shop and explains the various drugs. So when supplies are needed, the man travels on his motorbike to see his sister.

A larger pharmacy shop in the same market area is run by a Sino-Khmer couple, who also

2.1 Pharmacy shops are often family affairs.

do not have formal pharmacological education. The wife explains that vans from at least seven different companies call at the town about once a week. They deliver direct if they have the goods in the van; otherwise, the shopkeepers complete order lists, and delivery is made the following visit. This is a very convenient arrangement: until a year ago the woman had to go to Phnom Penh for supplies, but now she saves time and money for transportation, and can concentrate on running the shop, that also offers intravenous drips for rehydration and vitamin injections. She buys supplies from several companies: both Indian and Malaysian products are popular since they are relatively inexpensive. Many pharmacy owners tend to buy from only one or a few companies, preferably those that offer a discount or free samples on large orders, or reward orders over a certain amount with gifts like T-shirts, electric fans or rice cookers.

The distribution of pharmaceuticals by companies themselves began in the late 1990s, as main roads were improved and travel became safer. There were no longer attacks by remnant Khmer Rouge groups, and checkpoints, manned by demobilised soldiers who exhorted money from travellers, were abolished. Earlier, rural pharmacies had to fetch their supplies from larger pharmacies in Phnom Penh or the provincial towns, but they are now supplied by air-conditioned vans direct from the companies. This means that larger private pharmacies are now bypassed as suppliers, and control of the market has shifted to the companies. Only rather remote and/or small pharmacies are still supplied by larger provincial ones.

Neither the companies nor larger pharmacies are obliged to sell only to licensed shops, but ministry control at least implies a better chance that only registered drugs are distributed. The problem of counterfeit or substandard drugs is considerable. According to a recent study (Ministry of Health 2001), 13 percent of all drugs found on the market are counterfeit or substandard; the percentage among registered drugs was only 5.2, while among unregistered drugs it was 20.9.[7] By far the largest proportion of counterfeit and substandard drugs was found in unlicensed shops in the countryside, which is where the majority, and the poorest part of the population, get their supplies. The MoH study notes that none of the substandard or counterfeit drugs was domestically produced. Most customers, however, whether literate or not, still tend to believe that foreign drugs are better than those produced in Cambodia, because originally most imported drugs were French. Today, the unregistered drugs most likely to be fake come from other Asian countries, but they are still foreign (and therefore desirable), and they are often the cheapest.

Attitudes towards pharmaceuticals

The recent realisation by the Cambodian medical authorities that pharmaceuticals may be harmful (when substandard or counterfeit) has long been common knowledge in the premodern medical world in which healing and sorcery are two sides of the same coin. This attitude pertains equally to indigenous remedies and modern pharmaceuticals. When explaining his business of selling herbal medicine in the market, a herbalist emphasised that 'medicine is a weapon with two faces, it can kill or cure, heal or harm', implying that the beneficial or harmful effects depended on the provider.

The idea that the sale of some medical products should be restricted to customers with a prescription from a physician is foreign to almost everybody today, even though it is reported that, in the 1960s and 1970s, only over-the-counter drugs could be bought without a prescription (Gollogly 2002: 793). This does not mean it is immaterial to have a piece of paper with the name of a pharmaceutical product written on it. On the contrary, such slips of paper are highly valued, for both practical and conceptual reasons. Practically, it is convenient to have the name of a product written down in case you need it again; even if you cannot read it yourself, pharmacy shopkeepers can read it, and they will be able to dispense the right product quickly without engaging in a long conversation about symptoms and the like.

Conceptually, having the name in writing represents a certain sense of 'knowledge', but equally important, it is also magical. The efficacious principle of magic rests on the conflation of signifier and signified: for the illiterate customer, the possession of a slip of paper with an incomprehensible name, in an unfamiliar alphabet, inspires the same sense of confidence as magic charms and amulets; clutching such a slip of paper (together with a handful of Riels) is more than half the way to securing the product itself from the hundreds of equally exotic-sounding alternatives at the pharmacy. A common complaint is that customers only rarely get written names on the small quantities of different pills they purchase. Indeed, when we do exit interviews with pharmacy customers, they often ask us to write down the names of the products they have purchased. This complaint may also be interpreted as a complaint on a more profound level, namely that the patient/client is denied his or her active role in the healing process, by not being 'taught', rather than just receiving the curative substances.

Another customer expectation, which in contrast is almost always met, is the dispensing of several kinds of medicine, no matter what condition is to be treated. This idea also guides the practices of traditional herbalists (*kru khmer*), whose decoctions are made from a variety of herbal ingredients. Herbalists engage in 'mixing medicines' (*phsom thnam*), and the more ingredients they add, the greater their knowledge and reputation. The same idea is applied to pharmacy shopkeepers, known as *kru pet phsom thnam* ('teacher-medic mix medicine').

The pharmacy is in one sense representative of medical modernity, but in local practice it becomes synthesised with the premodern medical world. Although they sell biomedical pharmaceuticals, many pharmacy shopkeepers diagnose client conditions and dispense medicines according to notions derived from Ayurvedic principles. An important principle is the unobstructed flow of fluids, matter and wind through the conduits (*sasay*, which include blood-vessels, nerves, and tendons) in the body. A common cause of ailments is the blocking or jam-

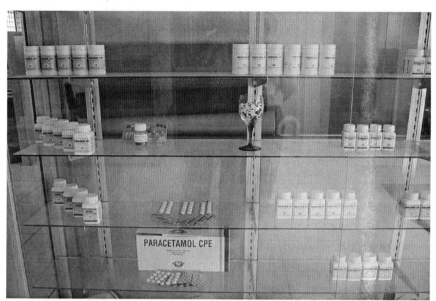

2.2 A leading domestic pharmaceutical company proudly displays its products in the reception area. The centrepiece 'cocktail' reflects the idea of mixing medicines.

ming (*stea*) of these conduits, and in most pharmacies one finds a prepared mix of remedies to unblock the flow: little transparent bags containing a couple of sedatives, antibiotics, painkillers and vitamins, each in a distinctive colour. Many people incur such blocking during the arduous working week; they need the medication to re-establish the flow over the weekend.[8] For other conditions, the shopkeeper also will provide a culturally suitable mix of products, preferably of different colours. Thus, if an antibiotic and a painkiller are indicated, he may double both – for example, giving both amoxicillin and ampicillin, and paracetamol and aspirin – throwing in a couple of different vitamin B and C preparations for good measure.

One unfortunate effect of this cultural expectation is that the small amount of money most customers have at their disposal will be spread over many non-essential products. When many people, for example, cannot afford a full dose of antibiotics, it does not improve things if they also have to spend money on biomedically unwarranted products. It becomes even worse when the supplementary products include potentially harmful drugs, such as corticosteroids that are increasingly popular among doctors, pharmacy shopkeepers and their clients.[9] Another effect of the demand for 'mixing' is that the market is flooded with numerous products containing the same formulae and differing only in brand name and price.

Pharmacists without pharmacies: the professionals

The risks that patients run at the pharmacy, by getting insufficient doses or even potentially harmful drugs, are exacerbated by the unregulated market for pharmaceuticals, and by the consequent growth in fake or substandard drugs. Of the many people who sell pharmaceuticals, trained pharmacists represent only a tiny proportion. Among them, an even smaller group works actively for their professional identity and the increased recognition of the pharmacy profession. In contrast to a mere occupation, a profession carries 'connotations of disinterested dedication and learning' which may be used to legitimate 'the effort to gain protection from competition in the labor market' (Freidson 1994: 18).

Not surprisingly, professionally committed pharmacists direct much of their attention to the competition from their rival profession, the physicians. According to the President of the Pharmacist Association of Cambodia, a major problem is that many government-employed physicians not only run a private clinic on the side, but have a pharmacy attached to the clinic, often run by the doctor's wife. Because of the higher status of the medical profession, the authorities turn a blind eye to the fact that strictly speaking, only professional pharmacists (and not physicians) may have a pharmacy license. Such physicians may augment their salary not only from their private practice but also from the substantial bonuses paid to them by certain pharmaceutical companies.

The Pharmacist Association currently has almost 600 members, about 95 percent of all active, professionally trained pharmacists in the country. By contrast, the Medical Association – as the President of the Pharmacist Association notes with some satisfaction – has only about 10 percent of eligible physicians as members. A more serious problem than competition from physicians is that only about 5 percent of professional pharmacists have their own pharmacy, despite several thousand pharmacies in the country. This paradoxical situation of having many pharmacists without a pharmacy, and an even larger number of pharmacies without pharmacists, is caused by historical particularities. After 1979 there were only a couple of dozen professional pharmacists in the country; of those who were students abroad before 1975 (primarily in France), virtually none returned, neither during Pol Pot nor during PRK, and the majority of already educated pharmacists had perished under Pol Pot. The first of the new generation graduated in the late 1980s, but by then the trade in pharmaceuticals was already dominated by non-educated business people. Some of these traders secured their urban property in 1979, when people were allowed to return to the cities and houses were up for grabs (because many of their previous inhabitants died under Pol Pot). Others invested their savings from the pharmaceutical trade in property around 1994, when the government banned the trade in pharmaceuticals from ordinary markets. In contrast, very few pharmacy students had the financial resources to set up a place of their own. Some pharmacists are employed in production, research, or development by domestic pharmaceutical companies; others take out a license and lease it to non-educated pharmacy owners.

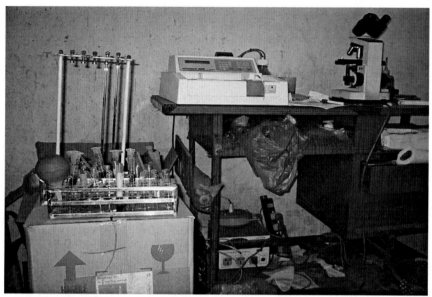

2.3 The private laboratory of a qualified pharmacist.

For a couple of newly graduated pharmacists with whom we spoke, the situation appeared rather bleak for them and their colleagues. During their studies, their identity had been formed through learning high professional standards, and thus the work conditions in real life came as something of a shock. Available jobs are mostly as sales representatives for foreign pharmaceutical companies (an option also open to newly graduated physicians), which require uncomfortable compromises with their identity and professional ethics. Few stay with such a job for long, and many leave the profession altogether.

Aspects of the situation for older professionals may be illustrated by the following case:

> Hang Luong is a pharmacist, currently director of a domestic (French-Cambodian) pharmaceutical company in Phnom Penh. He began pharmaceutical studies at the university in 1971 and was in his final year when the Khmer Rouge invaded the city in 1975. He and his brother were sent for compulsory manual labour in Kampong Cham province where the regime was relatively lenient; his mother and sister and a cousin were sent somewhere else, and he never saw them again. He returned to the capital in January 1979 and volunteered to work in the major pharmaceutical factory (presently called CPE, Cambodian Pharmaceutical Enterprises). He saw evidence that the Khmer Rouge had used the factory in their own way; jars of placenta in alcohol (used as fortifying tonic) were among the articles left on the shelves. He enrolled at the medical faculty as soon as it reopened in 1980, finished his education the following year, and continued working at the CPE. In 1985 the factory was temporarily closed and Luong was ordered to serve as the personal pharmacist (a kind of 'medical bodyguard') for the highest leadership of the party, including Heng Samrin, Chea Sim and Hun Sen. In

1993 he resigned from all his public duties, because he wanted to have no more to do with politics, and took a job doing blood tests at the Calmette hospital laboratory. He was among the first to do HIV tests and to call attention to the rapid spread of the virus. In 1996 he was offered a job at his present company; in the beginning they sold only five products, painkillers and antibiotics, but now they produce more than 70. They produce mainly for the domestic private sector – as the (now reconstructed) CPE has most of the contracts with the Ministry of Health for the public sector – but they also have modest exports to Vietnam and Togo. At the company, Mr Luong now places less emphasis on increasing production or market share, concentrating instead on quality control, which he sees as a professional responsibility that few other people take seriously. Apart from his company duties he lectures at the medical faculty, and he still does blood tests at Calmette. Formally it is the responsibility of the physicians to give patients the results of their HIV tests, but many shrink from this, so Mr Luong feels he has to take on this duty instead. This is not something he is happy about, as sometimes people kill themselves after getting the result. Mr Luong has not encouraged his children to become pharmacists; he sees it as a demanding profession with heavy responsibilities.

Pharmacies without pharmacists: the business people

As we have noted, the majority of pharmacy operators are non-professionally educated shopkeepers who trade in pharmaceuticals to make a living. Many entered this business in the dynamic situation following the Vietnamese invasion in 1979. The case of Ta Heang is in many ways typical:

Ta Heang is in his late fifties (Ta is an honorific meaning 'grandfather'); he owns a pharmacy in a provincial town. His father was a Chinese petty trader, his mother Khmer. As a small boy he often visited a playmate whose father had a pharmacy. Heang was absolutely fascinated with all the medical products he saw: with all the different bright colours they looked like candy. If only he could have afforded to study he would have become a pharmacist. Instead he learnt to do business from his father. During Pol Pot he was sent to do slave labour in the countryside with a mobile construction unit. One day his group was called to a meeting, where they received new clothes along with the information that they would be taken to another work site. As they walked along the road in the splendid new clothes and blue *kramas* (scarves), he met an old man who looked at him, admiring the new outfit, and seemed particularly fond of the *krama*. As in a vision he suddenly understood: one *krama*, one life. The new clothes made the people stand out and he realised that they were all to be taken away and killed. The old man said that he wouldn't mind exchanging his own worn *krama* for the new one; it was an offer to replace him. They exchanged their *kramas* and shirts. Heang continued to work as they arrived at the new destination and nothing happened to him. All the others in his group disappeared. It seemed to him that the old man on the road knew that the new *kramas* were a sign to the Khmer Rouge cadres, that he had deliberately saved his life by suggesting they exchange clothes. Heang never knew what happened to the old man but he decided to try and make his new life worthwhile. In

1979 he started with a little gold and entered the rice/pharmaceuticals trade in his home town of Kampong Chhnang, and as a skilful businessman, he was soon able to expand his pharmaceutical business. After plying his trade at half a dozen stalls in various markets – constantly forced to move by the authorities – he was able to buy a house with a shop near one of the main markets in 1995. For the past three or four years he has had a license, leased from a pharmacist for 100 USD per month; he also has to pay about 10 USD per month as tax to the government. He finds this a bit unfair since drug sellers without a pharmacy license can get away with paying only 500 USD a year (presumably to the local authorities). Very few of Ta Heang's clients come with a prescription. Ta Heang explains that most physicians make a deal with the pharmacy shopkeepers, offering to direct their patients to a particular shop, in exchange for 20 percent of the proceeds. Ta Heang refuses such deals, even if it results in fewer customers: it would mean raising prices, which he believes is unethical. Most of his clients are poor people, many ethnic Vietnamese (fisher folk) from across the river, or from the nearest floating villages on the Tonle Sap. Ta Heang often recommends Chinese herbal medicine (mostly in the form of pills, packed in bottles like biochemical products), because they may be a cheaper alternative. These products also have become more popular lately, he explains, because they do not create resistance like antibiotics. Ta Heang's concern for his clients' well-being also extends to sexually transmitted diseases: condoms are prominently displayed in his shop – something that attracts customers – and he is proud that he sells the cheapest condoms in town.

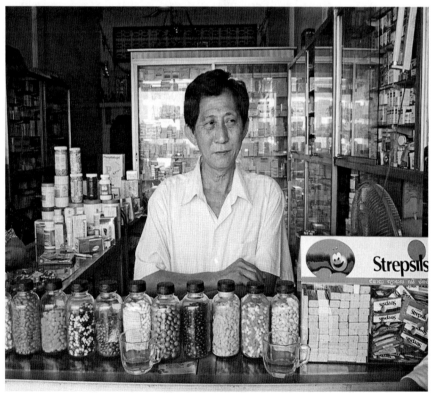

2.4 A proud shopkeeper in his well-stocked licenced pharmacy.

In contrast to a number of other pharmacy operators, Ta Heang was not adverse to our spending time in his pharmacy, observing the trade and asking details of the customers about their purchases, symptoms and treatment histories. In another provincial capital, we were turned away from several larger pharmacies, and our Cambodian assistants were intimidated when they attempted to do exit interviews with customers. We mentioned this to Mr Bun Savuth, deputy director of a provincial health centre, who was not surprised. The provincial drug inspection committee, of which he was chairman, had lately managed to reduce the number of illegal pharmacies/drugsellers around the central market from twenty to six. However, with the upcoming local elections (to take place in July 2003) there was no scope for further action, as the governor and other officials running for re-election were not disposed to initiate any measures that might disrupt their relations with important people in the electorate. The committee also had been unable to enforce the rule that licenced pharmacies may only sell pharmaceuticals; most also offer currency exchange and sell amulets, jewellery, cosmetics and shampoo, all 'magic' articles that, in the popular worldview, are included in the sphere of health, wealth and beauty.

Mr Savuth gave an example of one of the largest pharmacies in the city (to which we had been vigorously denied research access); it was owned by a big businessman whose fortune had been built on trans-border trade (i.e., smuggling) with Thailand. The main export article was gemstones, primarily in exchange for second-hand cars and pharmaceuticals. As the gemstone deposits became depleted, the merchant began dealing in rice, and he was now chairman of the provincial branch of the rice-millers' association; in that capacity he was recently Cambodia's representative at an international rice-producing conference in Singapore, with all expenses paid by the UNDP as part of an agricultural development programme. His shady business activities are wellknown, but the authorities cannot touch him. Another problem, according to Mr Savuth, is that the companies do not comply with the law. Instead of paying taxes to the government, they bribe the auditors and reward large customers with desirable gifts such as a motorbike for a purchase worth 10,000 USD. He does not place blame for the entire situation on anyone in particular, but concludes that if you abide by the law, you cannot be a businessman in Cambodia.

The rural practitioners

People in the countryside do not generally frequent district clinics or commune health centres. As we have mentioned, a nearby pharmacy or a village medic (*pet phum*) is normally the first choice. Such people often have rudimentary medical training, acquired either before or after Pol Pot, while some are uneducated ex-Khmer Rouge medics who rely on their treatment experience during Pol Pot. All of them engage in medicine to make a living, but as part of that identity most do it with a genuine sense of humanitarian responsibility.

While we were visiting Ta Heang's pharmacy, as described above, three Vietnamese people from a distant floating village on the Tonle Sap came in with a long 'prescription'; it was obvious from the number of products that the purchase was not for their personal use. Ta Heang explained that they were buying for a Vietnamese doctor who had settled in the village the past month. We decided to follow up the case and the next day we made our way, by car and boat to the village.

We boarded the houseboat of doctor Ngo Tang Ti just as the family was finishing a meal. The doctor welcomed us kindly, but was reluctant to talk about his medical practice; he was apparently rather frightened about our visit. His wife, on the other hand, became quite agitated; she complained loudly about the continual harassment by the Cambodian authorities of the Vietnamese in general, and of her husband in particular. In rapid succession she stuck under our noses an impressive number of papers: licences, passports, identity cards and the like, all the time insisting that her husband was doing nothing wrong. But, she said, the Khmer would probably come to kill them all, as they had tried before. We repeatedly explained that we did not work for the government, nor were we out to nail her husband in any way; and when the lady calmed down a bit, we talked to doctor Ti.

Far from being a recent arrival, the doctor had been living in the floating village since 1981. In 1983 Khmer Rouge soldiers had poured petrol over the houses and burnt the whole village. The family escaped by swimming ashore and hiding in the forest. Several people died and many were injured. The doctor was now 68 years old, had been in the Vietnamese army since the early 1950s, and he finished training as an army surgeon in 1958. He had come to Cambodia with the Vietnamese troops in 1979 and had retired two years later. He began by claiming that he no longer practised medicine; the government did not allow Vietnamese doctors to practise, and besides he had not renewed his licence (which was for doing 'mobile business' as a pharmacist, i.e., practising in the floating village). According to the rules, he was not even allowed to do emergency treatment or to treat his own family. The two medical cabinets in the room, however, told a different story, and he related how difficult it was for the villagers to reach the commune health centre ashore. Most of the time, moreover, there was nobody at the health centre; then people had to go all the way to the district clinic, which took a long time and cost money for transport. Sometimes, the commune health centre held courses or workshops for local medical personnel, but he was not allowed to attend because he was Vietnamese (or perhaps because his license had lapsed). Some Vietnamese practitioners would occasionally bribe the authorities to attend courses because they, too, needed the new knowledge.

While we were talking, another boat called at the house and a young mother brought in a two-year old baby who had suffered an accident. The mother had been chopping coconuts and the boy had managed to get his hand too close to the chopping board; his index finger had been split lengthwise. The doctor's wife immediately went into action, producing bandages, iodine, instruments on a tray, and a plastic basin of hot water. Meanwhile, doctor Ti tried to ignore the scene and continued talking to us. We suggested he had better attend to his patient, and with great relief he immediately did so, disinfected his hands and went to work. The cut in the baby's finger was quite serious and the wound was bleeding profusely. The doctor gave two injections (painkiller and anesthetic, presumably), cleaned and stitched the wound; it might not be state-of-the-art finger surgery, but preferable to going by boat all the way to the health centre, where the competence would probably not have been greater, and the kindness of the reception certainly less. After bandaging, the baby had a tetanus shot. Doctor Ti prepared three doses of pills, *para* (paracetamol), *ampi* (ampicillin) and Baralgine, plus a couple of unidentified pills from a large plastic jar, probably aspirin. The mother and baby left with her father who had taken them in his boat to the doctor. Now that we had seen the doctor in action, there was no more pretense, and he was visibly more at ease. We asked for the price of the treatment; it was 15,000 Riels (just under 4 USD), to be paid later. We said that as the woman was probably poor, it would be a pity if she should incur this extra expenditure, and so we paid doctor Ti on her behalf. He eventually accepted, gratefully and with immense relief. As we had in this way made ourselves complicit to the illegal treatment, even his wife became completely transformed at this gesture, and we took our leave as valued visitors.

Having seen the condition of medical services in this isolated community, we thought kindly of Ta Heang who had covered for his colleague (by implying that as a newcomer he had not yet managed a license). Later on we thought of the baby when we learned that Baralgine was a rather dangerous drug that had several years earlier been retracted completely by the Ministry of Health.[10]

The *kru khmer*

Indigenous healers in Cambodia are collectively referred to as *kru khmer* ('Khmer teachers'). Within this category there are several specialisations: bonesetters (*kru bakbek*), herbalists (*kru phsom thnam*), diviners (*kru teay*); some specialise in procuring charms and love-magic (*kru sneh*), while others are sorcerers (*kru thmup*). As already mentioned, the element of 'teaching' in the treatment is important to all, and this is what distinguishes traditional practitioners, *kru*, from practitioners of biomedicine, *pet* (from the Sanskrit *bedya*), no matter the level of training and competence of the individual. The element of teaching pertains both to the training of the *kru* and to the idea that the client/patient enters into a student-teacher relationship with the practitioner through the consultation. The relation of the *kru khmer* to his individual teacher (*kru thom*, 'big teacher') is both practical and spiritual. A teacher becomes 'big' after his death, when his practical teaching ceases, and his student erects a shrine for him in his house; all healing practices are carried out in cooperation with the *kru thom*, through burning incense and saying a prayer in front of his shrine. One *kru khmer* we visited even had to inform his *kru thom* before we could take his photograph. The spiritual component of the healer-client relationship may be illustrated in the following case:

Sok Cheat is a *kru khmer* in a village in Battambang province. He is 46 years old and has been a *kru khmer* since he was 17; his teacher, Aim Neang, also lived in the village, and he died in 1984 at the age of 87. He has four former students who all live in America; one sells traditional Khmer medicine. One of Cheat's specialities is making and selling protective charms to be worn on a string around the waist; he teaches people to recite magic formulae for making the charms effective. He is also a bonesetter and treats abscesses with herbal medicine. Medicine for abscesses is a mixture of three ingredients: yeast (*mee*), honey, and burnt crushed mussel or snail shells (*kambau*). The mixture is applied with a pad of cotton and then bandaged. When the mixture dries, it is moistened with alcohol. It is kept moist for one day, after which the patient is better. For bone-setting he makes a mixture of five ingredients: sticky rice; a herb (*slab changvar*, *Plantago major*); jujube leaves (*trouy putrea*, *Zizyphus jujuba*); a grass (*smao cheng kras*, *Eleusine indica*); and yellow ginger (*panlei*, *Zingiber zerumbet*). The mixture is wrapped in bamboo around the broken limb; young people will be cured in a week, for older patients it takes a bit longer. This mixture is also kept moist with alcohol. He also cures stomach infections and typhoid fever; for the former he prepares leaves of *slek tradet* (*Vitis pentagona*) boiled with palm sugar and water, to be drunk once a day for seven days. For typhoid, he uses pounded leaves of water green (*trakuon*, *Ipomoea aquatica*) in coconut juice, also to be taken for seven days.[11]

Cheat is very meticulous about paying respect to and informing his teacher. Before treatment, the patient has to provide a token of respect to the teacher, the *prea pis nokar*, which consists of one areca nut, five betel leaves, five cigarettes, five incense sticks, five candles, five units of money (500 Riels or Thai Baht) and five yellow flowers, to be placed at the shrine. Treatment consists not only of the application of the herbal mixtures but, most importantly, of the accompanying prayer. The 'prayer' or magic formula to be uttered is called *sot balai* ('Pali prayer'), and consists of the repetition of the words *ek, merk, smang*; these words have to be repeated a specific number of times according to the day of the week.

Apart from the symbolic gift of the *prea pis nokar*, a *kru khmer* must not demand payment for his services but relies on the generosity of his clients; in that respect his identity and status in society are more like that of a monk than that of a doctor (cf. Martin 1983; Eisenbruch 1992). The *sot balai* forms part of the whole complex of magical (Brahmanic) practices known as *mon akum* (from the Sanskrit *mant*, 'mantra', and *agama*, 'holy text'). Even if the knowledge of herbalism may ultimately be derived from Ayurvedic principles, no systematic application, or indeed awareness, of such principles is discernible among contemporary practitioners. Traditional medical knowledge is, indeed, local knowledge, fragmented and personalised. Some elder *kru khmer* remark that as part of their training they studied medical texts on palm-leaf manuscripts in the temples, thus forming part of a regional tradition of learning and knowledge. Yet, virtually all scholarly and philosophical literature was destroyed under Pol Pot, and contemporary traditional practitioners must rely on the teachings of their individual teacher(s).

In addition to vegetable matter, animal parts (e.g., tiger bones, dried snakes or geckos, or boar's tusks) are used in indigenous magico-medical concoctions. Some herbalists, moreover, while still referring to themselves as *kru*, are unencumbered by the spiritual dimension of their art. The following case is an example of a herbalist whose identity and career were formed during the non-capitalist modernity of the 1970s and 1980s.

Seng Huon produces indigenous herbal medicine and sells both his products and the unprocessed ingredients from his shop in the main market in Kampong Chhnang town. He is now in his late sixties. His father was a medical doctor employed at the leprosy hospital in Takhmau (south of Phnom Penh) who also took an active interest in traditional medicine; as a boy Huon was sent out to collect medicinal herbs and was taught about their properties by his father. In the late 1950s, Huon trained as a medical attendant for three years at the Ket Melea hospital in Phnom Penh, where he continued to work until 1975. He managed to pass himself off as a traditional healer to the Khmer Rouge and he was sent to a collective in the forest to serve as healer, produce herbal medicine, and teach herbalism to the Khmer Rouge cadres. When he got out from the forest in 1979, he was going to leave the country, but the Vietnamese put him to work at the provincial hospital in Kampong Chhnang as a medical inspector and herbal medicine specialist. During the Vietnamese period the authorities put great store by the medical potential of indigenous herbalism, and he became an important figure. But as Western pharmaceuticals became increasingly available in the early 1990s, the official interest in herbalism declined. Both his fame and his salary dwindled, and eventually he quit government service and set up his shop. He is quite bitter about his fate and feels he has been let down, or even betrayed, by the government.

Among his products, various wine tonics (*sra thnam*) are popular; the best used to contain tiger bones or python, but nowadays such ingredients are expensive and hard to find. The tonics are bottled and have Seng Huon's photo on the label; they are mainly used against rheumatic ailments, and numerous customers stop by his shop for a fortifying tonic, sold at 200 Riels for a small glass. Another popular remedy is a tonic for post-partum mothers. The post-partum period is subject to great ritual attention in Cambodia, but apparently neglected by the pharmaceutical industry, so here is a niche for local practitioners. Among the raw ingredients, the anti-malarial remedy known as *krob sleng* ('poisonous seed') sells well; it is a seed (of *Strychnos nux vomica*), the size of a coin, the active ingredient of which is strychnine, so it has to be administered with care. To begin a cure, the patient takes one eighth of a seed for the first couple of days, and gradually increases the dose to one half. *Krob sleng* is resorted to by the poorest customers (typically Vietnamese fisher folk) who cannot afford other practitioners.

Even if Seng Huon perceives himself, and is perceived by others, to be a *kru khmer*, he differs markedly from the majority of his colleagues, illustrating further the diversity of identities amongst Cambodian practitioners. He may perhaps be described as a neo-traditionalist. He survived Pol Pot because his secular herbal knowledge was deemed useful, and he became important during PRK as a state-promoted 'traditional' herbalist whose outlook tallied with the nationalist ideology of the Vietnamese-backed government regarding beliefs in the future of a domestic medical production from indigenous herbs. He differs from typical *kru khmer* in that he never conducted a healing practice from his house, but practiced in 'modern' institutional settings (the Khmer Rouge collective, the PRK district hospital). He is now a member of a traditional healers' association that seeks to reinvigorate herbal medicine. Called 'Association des Guérisseurs Khmers d'Angkor pour la Recherche des Médicaments Traditionelles en Vue de Developpement', the name indicates both its claim to authenticity, invoking ancient traditions from the Angkor period, and its modernist ambition to seek support

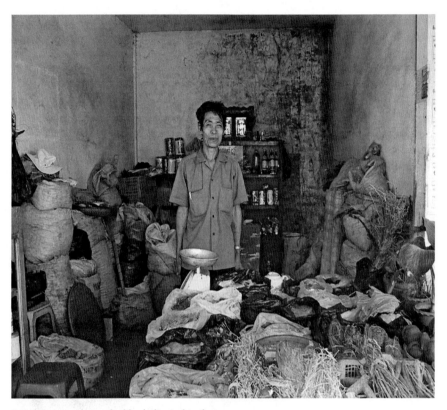

2.5 A 'neo-traditionalist' herbalist in his shop.

from international development organisations and NGOs (which have largely replaced government institutions as sources of legitimation and funding of development initiatives).

Conclusions: drug-providers, identity and modernity

In the above discussion of Cambodian medical identities, we have tentatively classified drug-providers into professionals, businesspeople, rural practitioners, and traditional healers, according to how they are positioned in regard to the distribution of medical substances. Among these providers, only the professionals may be said to have integrated into their identity the scientific worldview that the use of pharmaceuticals is assumed to presuppose. Perhaps most noteworthy about professional pharmacists as a collectivity, is their total lack of political power in Cambodian society. Within the context of the very weak government health system, along with the presence of development organisations, the relatively few pharmacists are easily marginalised by physicians, who are much more numerous. A tiny number of professional pharmacists struggle valiantly against the prevailing 'pharmaceutical anarchy' (Gollogly 2002: 793) by working for professional recognition, enforcement of the laws, good pharmacy practice, and drug quality control. The foreign pharmaceutical companies have little use for Cambodian pharmacists, and, paradoxically, only the smaller domestic ones can afford to keep employing someone like Hang Luong and allow him to slow down production for the sake of quality control. Among the younger qualified pharmacists, professional identity is rather fragile, and, as we saw, many recently qualified are likely to give it up altogether. In the case of pharmacists, the modernist idea of professionalisation is losing out to globalised capitalism in the a-modern Cambodian medical world.

The majority of the providers, the pharmacy shopkeepers who sell drugs to make a living, are cultural brokers at the interface between premodern customer expectations of magic and the modern pharmaceutical business. From this position they are able to transform and convert modern values by tapping into the premodern ones, but with the unintentional result that their customers often get the worst of both worlds, because of the shopkeepers' insufficient grasp of biomedical mechanics and their ready acquiescence to customer demands for 'mixing'. Nevertheless, the social identity of the majority of shopkeepers, as well as of the rural practitioners, is that of 'the poor man's doctor'. When Ta Heang, for example, was fortuitously given a new lease on life, he was able, because of his business acumen, to realise his boyhood dream of a 'candy shop', but in the process he also acquired a social conscience that makes him place concerns for the welfare of the poor above profit maximisation.

Yet, the individual and social identities of drug-providers are not shaped solely by their position in the provision system. An important factor in identity formation is the collective historical experiences of Cambodians during shifting political regimes, and their exposure to various degrees and versions of modernity and non-modernity. Common to almost all professionals and businesspeople, as well as most rural practitioners (above the age of about thirty) is their direct or indirect experience of the particularly vicious Pol Pot regime. Not belonging to the peasant class – which comprised more than 80 percent of the population – they were most likely classified as 'new people', of whom only about 20 percent survived the regime. Their exposure to the Khmer Rouge version of modernity thus implied an exceptionally dramatic rupture of what Giddens (1991) has called the 'protective cocoon' that safeguards a person's 'ontological security'. Likewise, the ontological insecurity of the Pol Pot regime did not quickly end with the demise of the Khmer Rouge; it persisted throughout the period of Vietnamese occupation and was in some ways compounded by the UNTAC intervention.

This ontological insecurity, we suggest, hit the professionals (qualified pharmacists as well as physicians) particularly hard. From having belonged to a celebrated intellectual elite of students during the post-independence period, they experienced total abjection under Pol Pot: their professional identity and competence was scorned and their human dignity assaulted.[12] Most elder professionals we have talked to have been adamant in insisting on their Khmer ethnic and national identity, through unsolicited declarations like 'I am Khmer and I stayed on Cambodian soil'. We interpret this insistence as a defence against possible allegations of un-Khmer dispositions; the Khmer chauvinism that attained extreme proportions under Pol Pot is still present in rudimentary form in the present-day political climate (cf. Ovesen and Trankell 2004). But during Pol Pot, even to be an urban dweller was un-Khmer, and the foreign medical or pharmaceutical education was seen as an affront against the indigenous Khmer medical tradition.

Paradoxically, the Pol Pot regime had pervasive consequences also for the traditional practices of indigenous healers. As already mentioned, written indigenous medical knowledge (on palm-leaf manuscripts) was largely destroyed, and spiritual teaching of students by healers was outlawed; those who kept up the spiritual aspect of their practices had to do so clandestinely and in isolation. The regime's assault on the whole tradition of spiritual teaching of indigenous healers, in which the client became affiliated to the 'line', or 'lineage' of the *kru* and his teacher(s), and in a way entered into the 'cult' of those teachers, was severely weakened. Nowadays, many indigenous practitioners follow the example of 'neo-traditional-

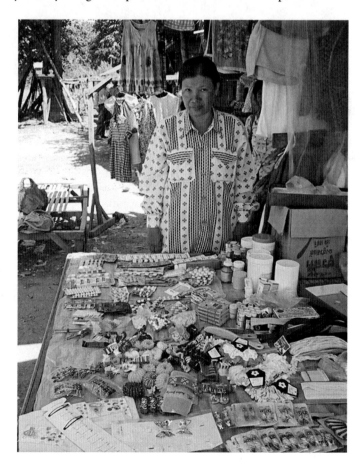

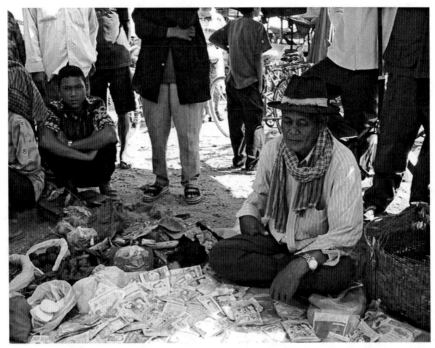

2.6, **2.7** The rural poor may find either pharmaceuticals or traditional remedies in the local markets.

ist' shopkeepers (like Seng Huon) and combine affiliation to the spiritual lineage with a commercialised customer relation, ephemeral and single-stranded.

From the perspective of medicinal consumers, the current situation is that many poor people cannot afford adequate biomedical treatment; indeed, what little medication they can afford is frequently either insufficient, substandard or superfluous. At the same time, because of the impoverishment of the indigenous *kru khmer* practices – in terms not only of spirituality but also of the insight and empathy generated through the diagnostic and healing process – the poor have reduced access to culturally, if not biomedically adequate, indigenous treatment which they would otherwise have been able to afford economically.

Despite the marked sense of social responsibility found in the majority of drug providers of all categories, and their honest intention to improve healthcare – not least among the poorer part of the population – these practitioners are to some extent unwitting hostages to the 'culture of indifference to affliction in an area of extreme inequality'. The reproduction of medical inequalities in the contemporary Cambodian a-modern medical world affects not only the health-seeking population but also the drug-providers.

Notes

1. This chapter forms part of a wider study on the indigenisation of modern medicine in Cambodia. Financial support from the Swedish Research Council is gratefully acknowledged. Fieldwork for this project has been carried out in periods between 1999 and 2004, following earlier field research since 1995. Among the several younger Cambodian colleagues who have participated in the project as research assistants and interpreters, we would particularly like to thank Heng Kimvan and Lath Poch. Names of informants mentioned in the text are pseudonyms.

2. In 2001 just over 90 percent of all pharmaceuticals in the country were imported; however, the value of these pharmaceutical imports was only 12 million USD (Ministry of Health 2001).

3. The country's leading hospital, the 'Russian Hospital' (a gift from the Soviet Union in the 1960s) in Phnom Penh, was mainly for treatment of the power elite, while the Calmette Hospital was reserved for children of the leadership.

4. Herbal medicine was traditionally taken as decoctions; a qualified pharmacist told us that the compression of herbs into tablets impeded the release of the active substances, and most of the 'rabbit shit' passed through the organism without having any effect whatsoever.

5. The Khmer Rouge abolished money, and gold became the main medium of exchange, even after money was officially reintroduced in 1981. Today, gold remains the preferred medium of exchange and standard of value for major economic transactions.

6. The figures are from a list compiled in 2001 by the Provincial Health Department; the list even includes the name of the owner and other particulars of each shop, something which no doubt facilitates the authorities' collection of the appropriate fees/fines for individual shops.

7. A national system of drug registration was introduced in 1994. Of the approximately 5,000 pharmaceutical products currently on the market, nearly 40 percent are unregistered; all unregistered drugs are (illegally) imported.

8. Sophisticated urbanites may instead go for novelties such as Kinal®, a mix of paracetamol and caffeine, marketed in white and blue packing for the busy executive and the housewife under stress respectively.

9. Corticosteroids are medically indicated for conditions such as asthma and arthritis. One of their effects is increased appetite and consequent weight gain, which is helpful for many clients. Other potential side effects, however, include restlessness, menstrual irregularities, insomnia, indigestion and peptic ulcers. Shopkeepers are not necessarily the main culprits here; a recent study (Rose et al. 2002) shows that physicians at private medical clinics in Phnom Penh routinely prescribe unnecessary corticosteroids.

10. According to the Vidal handbook of pharmaceuticals, Baralgine is a powerful analgesic to be used mainly in post-operative emergencies on (for example) severely traumatised soldiers on the battlefield. It should be used only when no alternatives are available, due to the high risk of haemorrhaging, which can cause shock and even death, regardless of blood transfusion. It seemed that the good doctor was relying on his old army surgeon routines.

11. The botanical names of the various remedies are in Douk Phana (1966).

12. 'To kill you is no loss, to keep you alive is no gain' was a slogan used by the Khmer Rouge about the 'new people' (Locard 1996).

References

Brun, P. 1998. *Cambodge. Médecine Traditionelle – Médecine Moderne: Lutte ou Confluence?* Thesis, Faculté d'Anthropologie et de Sociologie, Université Lumière Lyon II.

Chandler, D. 1993. *The Tragedy of Cambodian History.* South-East Asia ed, Chiang Mai: Silkworm Books.

Chhem, R. 2001. 'Les Doctrines médicales Khmères: Nosologie et méthodes diagnostiques'. *Siksacakr* (Siem Reap) 3: 12–15.

DeNike, H. et al. (eds). 2000. *Genocide in Cambodia. Documents from the Trial of Pol Pot and Ieng Sary.* Philadelphia: University of Pennsylvania Press.

Desbarats, J. 1995. *Prolific Survivors: Population Change in Cambodia 1975–1993.* Tempe: Arizona State University, Program for Southeast Asian Studies.

Douk Phana. 1966. *Contribution à l'étude des plantes médicinales du Cambodge.* Thesis, Pharmaceutical Faculty, Paris. Quimper: Imprimerie Ed. Ménez.

Eisenbruch, M. 1992. 'The Ritual Space of Patients and Traditional Healers in Cambodia'. *Bulletin de l'École Française d'Extrême-Orient,* 79, 2, 283–316.

Farmer, P. 2003. *Pathologies of Power. Health, Human Rights, and the New War on the Poor.* Berkeley: University of California Press.

Freidson, E. 1994. *Professionalism Reborn: Theory, Prophecy and Policy.* Oxford: Polity Press.

Giddens, A. 1991. *Modernity and Self-Identity: Self and Society in the Late Modern Age.* Oxford: Polity Press.

Gollogly, L. 2002. 'The Dilemmas of Aid: Cambodia 1992–2002'. *The Lancet,* 360, 9335, 793–8.

Hsu, E. 1999. *The Transmission of Chinese Medicine.* Cambridge: Cambridge University Press.

Locard, H. 1996. *Le 'Petit Livre Rouge' de Pol Pot.* Paris: L'Harmattan.

Marston, J. 2002. 'Democratic Kampuchea and the Idea of Modernity'. In *Cambodia Emerges from the Past: Eight Essays.* J. Ledgerwood (ed.), DeKalb: Northern Illinios University, Center for Southeast Asian Studies.

Martin, M.A. 1983. 'Eléments de médicine traditionelle khmère'. *Seksa Khmer* 6: 135–69.

——— 1994. *Cambodia: A Shattered Society.* Berkeley: University of California Press.

Ministry of Health. 2001. *Study Report on Counterfeit and Substandard Drugs in Cambodia 2001.* Phnom Penh: Ministry of Health & WHO.

Nguyen, V.-K. and K. Peschard. 2003. 'Anthropology, Inequality and Disease: A Review'. *Annual Review of Anthropology* 32: 447–74.

Ovesen, J. and I.-B. Trankell. 2004. 'Foreigners and Honorary Khmers: Ethnic Minorities in Cambodia'. In *Civilizing the Margins. Southeast Asian Government Programs for Development of Ethnic Minorities.* C. Duncan (ed.), Ithaca: Cornell University Press, pp. 241–69.

Piat, M. 1965. 'Médicine populaire au Cambodge'. *Bulletin de la Société des Études Indochinoises,* N. S. 40(4): 301–15.

Rose, G. et al. 2002. *Private Practitioners in Phnom Penh: A Mystery Client Study.* Phnom Penh: MoH, WHO, Options UK (mimeo).

Slocomb, M. 2003. *The People's Republic of Kampuchea 1979–1989: The Revolution after Pol Pot.* Chiang Mai: Silkworm Books.

Trankell, I.-B. 2003. 'Songs of Our Spirits: Possession and Historical Imagination among the Cham of Cambodia'. *Asian Ethnicity* 4(1): 31–46.

Trankell, I.-B. and J. Ovesen. 2004. 'French Colonial Medicine in Cambodia: Reflections of Governmentality'. *Anthropology and Medicine* 11(1): 91–105.

3

THE VICISSITUDES OF MEDICAL IDENTITY IN CAMEROON:

KEDJOM 'TRADITIONAL DOCTORS' AND AN AMBIVALENT CLIENTELE

Kent Maynard

As with any social definition of personhood, medical identity is created over time, collectively; individuals are never the sole authors of their identities. In this essay I consider so-called 'traditional doctors' in the chiefdom (or, more accurately, *fon*-dom) of Kedjom Keku in the Grassfields of the Republic of Cameroon.[1] In Pidgin English these men and women are called 'country doctors', in Ga'a Kedjom, *wu kɔfuh* (*ve mɔfuh*, pl.), or 'medicine person'. As I have argued elsewhere, *ve mɔfuh* do not pre-date European rule; indeed, they differ significantly from indigenous medicine (Maynard 2002; 2004). Appearing as early as the 1920s in towns, or as late as the 1950s in rural areas, the new healers are more professional and indivudualistic, more focused on intervention and somatic or psychiatric health care (than good or misfortune generally), and they are more commercial than indigenous medicine in the precolonial era.

In fact, healers pose challenges to the assertion and recognition of medical identity. Where indigenous medicine is firmly local, and grounded in the ritual arena, the country doctors attend to clients from their *fon*-dom and outsiders alike, often charging market prices. Lay Kedjom may have grave doubts about the legitimacy of such healers – and the veracity of their identity – especially because of their commercialism. At the same time, country doctors may try to mute such charges (and assert the authenticity of their identity as healers), by blurring the difference between commerce and ritual exchange. As a result, medical person-hood may follow a vexed career, first waxing and then waning precipitously.

Much of the Grassfields is in the Anglophone North West Province. Cameroon became a German colony in 1884; but with the First World War, it was divided between the British and French as a mandated trust territory until

1961.[2] Although the terrain can be rugged – and at 2,000 to 6,000 ft elevation – most groups produce a horticultural surplus and possess a formal political hierarchy. At the apex are two major political and ritual authorities: *kwyfon* is an umbrella association, subsuming an array of groups open to all initiated Kedjom men; alongside *kwyfon* is the *fon*, a hereditary ruler who is the key intermediary with the ancestral and spiritual afterworld. The *fon* and *kwyfon* carry out major political responsibilities, but have religious, medicinal, economic and other duties as well. For our purposes, *kwyfon* and the palace are principally responsible for promoting and renewing the welfare of the *fon*-dom, including health, reproductive welfare, and economic prosperity of the Kedjom people, their land, crops and animals.

Precolonial medicine bears little resemblance to the organisation and cultural ideology of the *ve mǝfuh* or country doctors, although their etiology, iconography and techniques may be similar. Put baldly, the usual English gloss for these healers as 'traditional doctors' is oxymoronic. *Ve mǝfuh* arose in light of multiple factors: new institutions introduced by European and mission authorities (including biomedicine), the rising tide of the market, and greater individualism. Responses to this new tradition remain ambivalent. Some Kedjom accept the legitimacy of the doctors but measure them against their own yardstick, the market principle of 'value for money:' i.e., have healers done what they claim to do? Others question the very premises of the new medical tradition and find it wanting. Because precolonial medicine was part of ritual exchange – quite distinct from what Kedjom see as the necessary evil of the market – to turn medicine into a business can in fact be quite threatening.

If lay people doubt the identity of the new healers – and this varies, as we shall see – they do so on two grounds. Some view them collectively as charlatans: what healers do is not medicine. Others see them as frauds on a case-by-case basis, for example, if an individual healer has too many failures. Either way, commercialism bears the brunt of blame: as people say, 'money spoils medicine'. The result is that healers may have careers, and an identity, fraught with vicissitudes. They may enjoy great popularity only to see their local clientele dwindle to virtually nothing.

Who is a 'traditional doctor'?

Let me begin with an illustration. Returning to Kedjom Keku in 1996 after an absence of six years meant that my wife and I were eager to see our many friends in the village. My wife lived first in Kedjom Keku, beginning in 1981, and had become good friends with a hard-working man (and his equally industrious wife) who generally spent his days as a yardman looking after the compound of an absentee landowner; but he also engaged in hunting, and a number of other small businesses along with his wife, to augment the family budget. Thus, we were intrigued to learn that 'Pa' now claimed that 'Gods' (*ve nyngong*, pl.; *nyngong*, sgl.)

had come to him in dreams, asking him to be a healer (*wu kɔfuh*).[3] Two rooms in his house were now given over to his newfound practice, with one table taken up entirely with an enormous array of herbal and other therapies that he used in treating patients. Old clay pots, leaves, half calabashes, horned cups, divining implements, and other arcane tools of his trade were arrayed neatly around his rooms. Stalks of *nkung*, a succulent associated with the Gods – because of its apparently miraculous powers to be cut, replanted, and to grow again, and essential to most rites – grew in and around the compound, along with the equally crucial camwood, ground, iridescent and red-orange. Behind his compound he pointed out a garden with a host of plants; 'these are my medicines', he told us proudly, but he also gathered additional ingredients on his many forays into the mountain forests, or the valleys choked with elephant grass that surround the village.

Pa told us that Gods, the *ve nyngong*, had visited him in dreams, to teach him the medicines and therapies for a variety of afflictions. Over time, they had given him more and more treatments as new problems cropped up in his patients. These included human ailments, but other difficulties as well; for example, he had recently treated a neighbour's car that refused to start. After first divining that a witch was attacking the neighbour through afflicting the car, Pa sacrificed a fowl, spraying its blood across the front bumper, and placing an animal skin bag filled with protective medicines carefully out of sight under the driver's seat.

What was especially intriguing is that Pa's identity as a healer or *wu kɔfuh* did not spring into existence all at once, fully formed. When my wife and I first knew him in 1981, he had already inherited several medicines from family members that he used in treating his family or a few friends or neighbours who might come to him. He spoke especially of medicine for menstrual cramps and 'belly bite' (gastro-intestinal disorders), as well as medicine to protect a person against witchcraft when they left the village (Susan Diduk, personal communication).[4] We might come upon him late in the afternoon cutting up plants gathered on a hunting trek into the mountains, drying the herbs in the sun on a woven grass tray, or grinding them in a pestle and mortar.

By 1989, Pa's medicinal practice had expanded. He was treating more patients and for money, and he had augmented his array of therapies by purchasing medicines (and the instructions for their use) from other 'traditional doctors' in the village. It was only by 1996, that he was also receiving medicinal knowledge from the Gods in dreams. He liked to receive his patients 'privately,' he said, 'like the doctors at Mbingo', a North American Baptist hospital seven miles away. A client would be ushered alone into a small room where Pa would diagnose the problem, often using an antelope horn rattle divining instrument. On being asked a question, the rattle (filled with stones and covered with skin) would either make noise or fall silent, confirming or refuting the query. If he did not already possess the proper medicinal treatment, Pa was confident that his patron Gods would reveal the remedy in the course of his dreams.

Ve Mɔ̀fuh and indigenous medicine

How should we interpret this? My friend has amassed, intentionally or not, a collection of objects that have long been identified with healing and the spiritual
realm. Likewise, divination, protective medicines against witchcraft, the use of
nkung, the sacrifice of fowls, and other practices, are all well known and rooted in
the precolonial past. There is no confusion among Pa's neighbours about who he
claims to be: a *wu kɔ̀fuh* or healer. Indeed, the symbols of his medical identity
enjoy wide consensus. *Ve mɔ̀fuh* vary in their iconography and practice, but his
particular objects and actions are not in doubt. For most Kedjom, the first question is one asked of any new doctor: Is this person what he or she claims to be? Is
he really a *wu kɔ̀fuh* or only pretending to heal? When a new healer arises through
dreams or visions, such as Pa, people may wonder if the person is 'sick'. After all,
the Gods may demand dietary restrictions and apprentice healers may lose
weight. Eccentric, or even antisocial behaviour, such as refusing to greet people or
to leave the compound, may also signal to lay Kedjom that the person is 'off-
senses' or mad. Still others may suggest rather cynically that the new healer is
doing this out of economic hardship; overwhelmed by debt the person has sought
another means of livelihood.

For some Kedjom, however, the training of someone like Pa is readily seen as
genuine. They recognise and accept the deeply held signs of the Gods or ancestors visiting the living in dreams or visions. People 'stolen' by the spirits are said
to *fentɔ*. Usually translated as 'transform', in Pa's case *fentɔ* means to 'move about
in dreams', or more corporally to be 'lost for bush', sometimes dragged by Gods
into pools for weeks or apocryphal years. During this time alone, the healer
receives training from the Gods, and returns to the village bearing the recognised
signs of healing, the *nkung* plant, camwood, or various herbs and stones.

People 'taken' by spirits, or those like Pa instructed to heal, are part of a long,
well-established claim in the Grassfields. Since *fentɔ* is extraordinary and powerful, it marks those it touches with strange signs, at times vexatious to people left
behind. All medicines have their own 'laws' (*ɔ̀sauh*) that, if transgressed, cause
misfortune or 'spoil' the efficacy of the medicine. Doctors like Pa also have laws,
and they must obey the God's instructions. Once people accept that a God or
ancestor has visited a person, they recognise that those so touched are not mad,
foolish or perverse. Rather, they act from an ethical imperative: for their health or
very lives, healers must obey the rules of their spiritual guides.

The social organisation of precolonial medicine

We see in Pa's experience something of the history of Grassfields' therapeutic life.
But it would be a mistake to equate what Pa does with precolonial medicine. Far
too briefly, let me sketch out indigenous medicine.[5] First, it was and is anchored
in groups. As Pa did in 1981, Kedjom men (as most women were ineligible) could

inherit knowledge, join medicinal houses or lodges, or receive medicine from the ancestors or Gods (as Pa was doing after 1996). But medicine was never bought or sold, nor was it more than a semi-speciality. Medicine people did not act alone; they formed medicinal societies, whether in the palace or individual compounds.

As with Kedjom society and the spiritual world, medicine was hierarchical, with the *fon* said to 'know' all medicine as a nominal or active member of all medicine houses. Indeed, all new medicines revealed by the ancestors or Gods had to be brought to the palace and shown to the *fon* and his group of priestly advisors (*vɔpfem*). At the apex, *kwyfon* subsumed three priestly societies in the palace: *vɔpfem* is charged with the care of royal ancestors and the most important Gods protecting the entire *fon*-dom, while *ngontoh* and *ngalim* are two major medicine houses (though there are or were many others). Each of these groups engaged in medicinal rites and/or sacrifices on fixed occasions in the ritual calendar, as well as in particular emergencies, such as polluting events like epidemics or during warfare, e.g., when enemies burn crops. Through sacrifices to the *ve nyngong* and ancestors, and the fortification of medicinal shrines encircling and doting the *fon*-dom, all these groups work to ensure Kedjom welfare. In addition to the palace houses, there are compound medicine houses performing essential rites for the entire society, e.g., the burial of witches, the disinterment of ancestral skulls or teeth, and so on. Finally, there are compound medicine houses devoted principally to the welfare of their members, whether problems of health, crop and household protection, economic prosperity and so on.[6] If one received medicine from the spirits in dreams, one was always instructed to form such medicine houses, with the God dictating who should be a member.

Indigenous medicine is in every sense local, meant only for the Kedjom. In the nineteenth century outsiders could not join any medicine house, nor could members received clients from other *fon*-doms. Medicinal knowledge is secret, not just from outsiders, but uninitiated Kedjom as well. Such secrets are acquired by joining the house via *tangɔ* – literally, 'to count' – a series of ritually stipulated gifts. Note the moral weight of secrecy: keeping the secret is necessary to the efficacy of the medicine and the welfare of the *fon*-dom (cf. Diduk 1987).

The professionalisation of 'traditional medicine'

All of this is changing. *Ve mɔfuh*, or the new 'country doctors', have been present in Kedjom from the late 1940s, but have increased greatly in numbers since the 1980s, both locally and in the Grassfields generally. As of 1998, there were about 40 healers in Kedjom Keku alone. Some receive medicine from Gods, others via purchase or apprenticeship, through dreams from ancestors or inheritance from a parent. In Pa's case, he has learned his medicine in all three ways, via inheritance, purchase and dreams. In any case, the proliferation of healers reflects the growing professionalisation of medicine across sub-Saharan Africa (Lantum 1985; Last and Chavunkuka 1986). In Cameroon, these new practitioners often seem adept at negotiating the commercial world. Healers practise alone, but some create elaborate 'herbal homes', compound-based clinics that resemble biomedical clinics in their organisation, and in the control exercised over patients and their bodies.[7] Signboards in urban and rural areas alike declare their specialities and *bona fides*, including their government licence to advertise. 'Wembah Daniel, Traditional Doctor', states a large sign on the major 'ring road' in the North West Province; and in Pidgin and local spelling it proclaims, 'Specialist in: Fractures, Dislocations, Poison, Dysentery, Veneral Disease, Dropsy, Whoping Cough [*sic*], Toothache, Dectator [*sic*] of Thieves, Phentinsick [*sic*] [i.e., 'fainting sick', or epilepsy]'.

Precolonial medicine had empirical consequences but, like all medicine, it was equally a moral enterprise. The social organisation of prevention and intervention reflect the larger drama between the forces of dissolution and those promoting welfare of the *fon*-dom. Medicine was not narrowly construed to be about somatic or psychiatric health; it was bound up instead with the promotion of group wellbeing and its protection from abomination, pollution, and misfortune broadly defined. What happens to this institutional ethics when medicine becomes a business transaction for the new healers, especially when *fon*-doms are 'dual principle' societies divided between ritual and market exchange (Rowlands 1987: 62–63)? Put another way: what becomes of medical identity when healers attempt to remove medicine from the ritual domain and make it a market transaction? Finally, and in light of this shift in domains, how do the healers construct their identity, and how do clients assess these efforts?

There have always been questions about the legitimacy of country doctors, or *ve mɔ̀fuh*, ever since they arose in Kedjom Keku in the 1940s, but these have grown more fractious with the economic difficulties of the last two decades. We cannot understand the terms of the debate, or its relevance for medical identity, without addressing a series of issues. First is the centrality of the market in the precolonial Grassfields, and the deep unease about its influence. The second is how the ethics of ritualised exchange, the giving of formal gifts in exchange for a wide variety of rights (whether to marry, join a host of groups, to display the special insignia of status, or so on) are related to these tensions. This group-centred ethic requires that profits gained at market be converted into the social capital of title-taking and polygyny. What might lead to individual aggrandisement ends up legitimating a hegemonic moral order that presupposes both hierarchy and central control over the economy and surplus wealth.[8]

The Kedjom 'moral polity'

To examine these issues let me begin with the concept of 'moral polity'.[9] If medicine before the German era was a moral act, this is no less true today. But where precolonial medicine is essential to *fon*-dom well-being, the new professionalised healers, and their identity, are morally ambivalent. While people certainly go to country doctors, they may suspect their motives and efficacy, and voice concern about their impact on Kedjom welfare. To understand this let me situate medicine in the moral economy or, better said, the 'moral polity' of Kedjom life. James Scott (1978) originally used the term 'moral economy' to argue that subsistence activities may bear a moral import that helps define peasant resistance to economic or political injustice. How people make a living epitomises a great deal about who they are, and more to the point, who they think they ought to be. When that sense of identity – our deepest sense of individual and social personhood – and the means of livelihood underlying it are endangered, it is more than just physically daunting: it is morally threatening as well.

The same is true with politics. As the past several years remind us, relationships between peoples or states are not simply a matter of *realpolitik*; politics propose and presuppose moral assumptions. The Kedjom are no exception. Jean-Pierre Warnier (1975) and Michael Rowlands (1987: 56) argue persuasively that we mistake the nature of Grassfields *fons* if we see them as primarily political. The *fon* did hold real power, exercising control over people and the economy, But the power of the *fon* was and is articulated through an elaborate moral discourse. It is he who shoulders the burden of coordinating relations between his subjects and the ancestral and Godly world for protection, prosperity and welfare. His authority rests on a primarily spiritual, moral, and medicinal identity bent wholly towards preserving and promoting the well-being of his *fon*-dom. Without his mediation, the very sovereignty of his *fon*-dom is at risk.

This ideology is not mere window dressing: it helped redirect potentially disruptive economic activities to bolster the social and political structures of the *fon*-dom. Precolonial Grassfields societies confronted a common economic paradox: they produced a surplus of some goods, but not others. Engaged in specialised trade –of ironware in Kedjom Keku, for example – they 'made market' for what they lacked. *Fon*-doms might need palm oil for cooking but they also required camwood and other ritual essentials. Cloth, glass beads or carved stools were also highly desirable, emblematic of rank and prestige.

Trade introduced a double tension into Grassfields societies. Internally, it meant that artisans (such as excellent carvers) and traders might amass sufficient wealth and control over labour to challenge the dominance of the royal clan and other elites (Rowlands 1987). Externally, it meant that *fon*-doms had to engage in trade for essential items, but with groups who might threaten their sovereignty. Control over trade routes and economic goods was a constant source of struggle in the nineteenth century, conflict that was exacerbated by the migration of new groups into the area, notably the Chamba and Fulani. In this rancorous context, medicine served to buttress the *fon*-dom against the threat of internal and external disorder. Medicinal institutions, the various priesthoods and their activities, were focused on the welfare of the *fon*-dom. In the process, they proclaimed and vouchsafed the legitimacy of political structures and their agents. Medicine is best defined as public well-being: it is carried out in groups for the protection of groups and the promotion of their welfare, whether for the compound, lineage, clan or *fon*-dom, or the myriad associations integral to Grassfields life.

Precolonial Kedjom medicine was firmly tied to the defense of the *fon*-dom; as a 'moral polity' the *fon*-dom itself was therapeutic, ensuring health, fertility and economic prosperity for the entire group.[10] But this implies that medicine is ideologically opposed to the market, with its twin threats of personal wealth and uneasy relations with other societies. Legitimate medicinal power is part of the hierarchical structure of Kedjom society. Its secrets are acquired through ritual gift giving, or *tangə*, by which aspirants gain title to ever more powerful and prestigious positions in society. In short, Kedjom ethics assume a split between the public, acceptable realm of medicine, ritual exchange and title-taking, versus the private, suspect nature of economic exchange, the necessary but fraught involvement in a regional economy.

This split and tension between ritual and market exchange pre-date European rule. Rowlands (1987: 61) and Warnier (1975: 322) argue for the presence of a mercantilist economy with standard currencies already in the seventeenth century; by the nineteenth century, trade gained an average profit of over 50 percent. The market and ritual arenas are so deeply entrenched, that Rowlands (1987: 62–3) calls groups in the Grassfields 'dual principle' societies. For Rowlands, ritual exchange is epitomised by bride service, and I would add *tangə*. It suggests a prestige economy, and a 'collectivist' ethic uniting 'a moral definition of authority with ritual practices ensuring group harmony and conflict resolution...' (1987: 63). In contrast, trade and especially slavery were redolent of turpitude. We can see why commerce might suggest witchery, 'bad medicine' (often translated as 'sorcery'), 'the unconstrained pursuit of power over others, the use of coercion and violence, and all forms of individualistic and selfish behaviour' (Rowlands 1987: 63).

Witchcraft and bad medicines are associated not just with commerce, but with marketplaces, where one frequently finds outsiders buying and selling.[11] The two main markets in Kedjom Keku have medicine shrines (*vəfam*) renewed seasonally by *ngalim*, a medicinal priesthood in the palace. By extension, even money can be suspect. Thus, one should never let it touch food; money has passed through the hands of many strangers. Who knows what they may have done to it?

Witches also are said to bring evil from outside the country. They join at market to buy and sell their evil goods and produce. Local witches can sell crops to 'foreign' witches so that Kedjom's crops will not flourish. Thus, witches prosper economically at the expense of individuals or the group. 'Witch markets' have many entrances as witches come from different ethnic groups. Kedjom men and women with the 'four-eyed', clairvoyant ability to see witchery and warn of its presence —collectively referred to as the 'eyes of *kwyfon*' (*əshə kwyfon*) – are said to station themselves outside these mystical markets, standing guard at vulnerable road junctions.

Given the association of markets with witchery, Kedjom unease about the new country doctors begins with the fact that they commodify medicine. But it also relates to selling medicine or knowledge to Kedjom and non-Kedjom alike. Even Europeans like myself can now apprentice with the new doctors or diviners, unheard of for medicine houses before colonialism.[12] Those allowed to participate in medicine defined the limits of Kedjom ethnic identity. Non-Kedjom, by definition, could not learn Kedjom medicinal secrets. Nor could one bring medicine into Kedjom from outside. Even the *fon* home from a trip was medicinally cleansed. The thought was that 'bad medicine' secretly placed on the *fon* by 'foreigners' could bring ruin to the palace, the medicinal and spiritual heart of Kedjom.

The ties between the market, foreignness, witchery and bad medicine are clearly related to economic rivalry and political expansion in the precolonial era. But the association of witchery and foreigners is also grounded in cosmology. There is no sense that Kedjom ever considered themselves to be uniquely or preeminently human. There is evidence, however, of separate creation stories for each *fon*-dom.[13] Likewise, Kedjom argue that their Gods and ancestors promote the welfare specifically of the Kedjom; the spiritual world does not aid or succour potential enemies.[14]

Bound to cosmology and *taŋɔ̃*, medicine, too, is indisputably local. Even the first of the new Kedjom country doctors did not sell medicine or treat clients in other villages. Just as other *fon*-doms would have objected to the introduction of 'strange' medicine, the Kedjom *fon* and *kwyfon* would not permit Kedjom medicine to be used for outsiders. The same objections hold true for compound medicine houses: their therapies are meant only for the Kedjom. There is absolutely no evidence from the nineteenth century that such houses received outsiders for treatment. It is even less likely that house members left the *fon*-dom to practice elsewhere; and certainly itinerating with medicine is unheard of for the precolonial era.[15]

This indigenous view of medicine, as Kedjom-specific, contrasts sharply with contemporary Kedjom healers who argue for the universal efficacy of medicine. The healer mentioned earlier, for example, does not itinerate with his medicine, but he will treat outsiders in his compound. Likewise, he once invited a young healer from Oku, another *fon*-dom, to live in his compound. Pa has one son who suffers from epilepsy: although Pa has treated him with local medicine, as well as phenobarbital from the North American Baptist Hospital at Mbingo, he also asked the other healer to treat him as well.

All country doctors of whom I am aware claim their therapies are appropriate for anyone, whether they are from their *fon*-dom or not. At times, they justify their claims of universality through appeals to Christianity. I once visited a well-respected healer who was also Catholic. He noticed that I had begun to use reading glasses, and without my prompting he consulted his God (speaking in tongues) to report that a witch in the US was 'spoiling' my eyes out of jealousy. I should seek treatment from him as his medicine would be just as effective for me as for the Kedjom. We humans, he said, are 'all one'. Regardless of 'race' we are 'all brothers'. There is only 'one God' and 'Adám and Eva' are ancestors for all of us.

Tangə̀ ə̀sho and the moral challenge of the market

I do not want to exaggerate the opposition either between commerce and ritual, or between external sources of evil and internal harmony. In the Grassfields there were a variety of ways to bring commercial and political relations with outsiders within the ritual pale; so too witchcraft and bad medicine could originate with kin and neighbours, not just outsiders.[16] Yet, *fon*-doms have long had to contend with dilemmas caused or exacerbated by surplus production and external trade. Given the social ethic, focused on the importance of the group, individuals should not be arrogant simply because they have money. Yet wealth is inevitable from trade and the market; what should they do with their newfound profit? Title taking and polygyny, and other aspects of the prestige economy, were the only morally palatable alternatives. If traders did not redistribute wealth, by taking wives or titles, they risked censure. *Kwyfon* and the palace might send masquer-aders to destroy the possessions of haughty men who had grown rich through trading, but who refused to take titles (Rowlands 1987: 62).

Title taking, marriage and the insignia of prestige all involve *tangə̀* and ritual exchange. *Tangə̀* means 'to count' and 'to greet' (or, in Pidgin, 'to salute'). The term *ə̀sho* in Ga'a Kedjom refers to rank or position. *Tangə̀ ə̀sho* is 'to count rank' or 'salute one's status'.[17] One must *tangə̀* to receive any title or cultural privilege – e.g., a woman's right to see her grandchild or a man's to sit on a particular kind of carved stool – or to enter the various medicinal groups and other lodges of Kedjom society. This is true across the Grassfields; thus, in Mankon, *tsama* means to give to those who have already gained the right to bestow privileges (Warnier 1975: 160). Once acquired, of course, these new titles garner power to gain other privileges, including more wealth. Note how this helps define the moral charac-ter of wealth. Money alone does not denote evil, selfishness or avarice (though it can pollute). In fact, without wealth or privileges a person counts for little. But to be ethically above board, wealth must be acquired via *tangə̀ ə̀sho*. Not wealth *per se*, but wealth gained from commerce – and then hoarded or reinvested only in the market – is considered immoral. On the other hand, to acquire wealth, spend it on '*tsama*-able' privileges to gain prestige, power and more wealth, is entirely laudable.[18]

Whether we speak of people, land, medicine or food (with a few exceptions), these should not be treated as commodities.[19] Historically, there were fewer mar-kets in the Grassfields, and they were highly regulated by ritual restrictions. Some items were simply excluded from sale, including subsistence crops and medi-cine.[20] Kedjom still do not use the terms 'sell' (*zen*) or 'buy' (*batlə̀*) in regard to medicine or medicinal knowledge. Patients receive (*she*) local medicine and give (*kuh*) something in return. And, all new members of a medicine society, must '*tangə̀* the house' through fixed gifts, such as goats, fowls, vegetable food, corn beer, palm oil and/or other items.

At times, *tangə̀* is said to be like 'marriage', ideally permanent and with ongo-ing obligations (cf. Diduk and Maynard 2001). Each medicine house – indeed, each medicine – has its own 'law' (*∂sauh*), magical and morally charged prescriptive behaviours in regard to the medicine and towards other members of the house. Foremost is the need to be of 'one heart', to act without anger, jealousy or malice. There should be no deception, theft, or adultery between members or their families. When the Kedjom say that medicine is 'free' they do not mean people give nothing to acquire it; rather, they are pointing to a fundamental difference between ritual and the market. The latter underscores the principles of supply and demand, whereas ritual assumes invariance in the terms of exchange. It does not matter if there is high demand for medicine against fever, or that fewer people wish to join a particular medicine house. What one gives, as people say, should not change by 'one red franc' or one fowl from its medicinal law. To change the gift, to turn *tangɔ* into a purchase, dissipates medicinal power and risks calamity for the seller.[21]

Commercialisation and medical identities

Europeans did not introduce markets or trade, but commercial enterprise increased significantly with German and British rule. There is a deep and increasing sense of moral corruption in the Grassfields, especially with the last two decades of economic difficulties. When commerce threatens to take over medicine what happens to therapeutic institutions and the identity of their practitioners? People are divided in their response. Kedjom go to country doctors but are leery of commercialism. Scepticism and even cynicism about the healers or *ve mɔ̀fuh* has increased with the 'economic crisis'. Practitioners like Pa, whose story is recounted above, may come in for criticism given the unseemly coincidence of their increased medicinal practice precisely when there is deepening economic stagnation. Indeed, although Pa continues to practise, relatively few Kedjom clients seek him out.

In fact, we can see a continuum from the least to the most commercial healers reflecting Kedjom ambivalence. When country doctors go too far, too blatantly selling medicine, it invites censure. As Irving Goffman (1963) remarked in a different context, they risk 'spoiling' their identity, losing their legitimacy and instead being identified as 'quacks' or 'charlatans'. As a result, some country doctors emulate the individualistic and market aspects of biomedicine, while others resist or blur them. The new medicine remains a contested arena between practitioners who vary in their commitment to *tangɔ*. Who gains the upper hand, and what Grassfields medicinal identities will look like in the future, remain unresolved.

While all Kedjom healers whom I know are open to treating 'foreign' patients, they are not equally commercial. Lay Kedjom commonly suggest that some country doctors are more 'money-minded' than others; likewise, some healers more than others acknowledge that they engage in business. In the Grassfields generally, some healers charge up front, regardless of success; others charge after the event and only if therapy is successful. Still others do not charge at all, relying instead on gifts. In yet further variations, some healers accept gifts for some treatments while charging for others, or charge some clients but not others.

Blurring commercialism

In describing the ambivalence of the commercial sphere, I do not mean that the mere act of going to market casts a suspicion of witchery. Witches 'make market', but when people buy or sell they emphatically are not making witchcraft. This applies equally to the new country doctors. People may suspect that the most commercial healers are fraudulent, but they never say that such healing is witch-craft; nor is the identity of the new healers associated with witchery. The point is that commerce is morally devalued, or a necessary but risky endeavour. Trade may be unavoidable, but if it disrupts the moral polity, it threatens the welfare of the *fon*-dom.

How do country doctors respond to the moral ambiguity of their practice, and to the scepticism of potential clients? How do they address these misgivings about or outright critiques of their identity as healers? They are clearly aware of the widespread discourse that suspects (some of) them of quackery, or ruining their medicine through avarice. Traditional doctors' associations in urban areas may issue declarations condemning quackery (Ngwa 1998; Shiyntum 1998). Nor is it surprising that healers resemble the lay public in associating charlatanism with the more commercial practitioners. A member of the traditional doctors' association in the South West Province noted in a newspaper interview that, '[t]he lack of employment opportunities today had pushed so many people to become tradi-tional practitioners, it is regrettable and catastrophic' (Ngalame 1998: 7). The Association also 'condemned money-making and [the] get-rich-quick-attitude of some of their colleagues who advertised their prowess through signboards [or] radio messages' (1998: 7).

In Kedjom, a common stance of the new country doctors (whether conscious or not) is to blur or deny the charge of being commercial. One healer argues that she has no choice but to itinerate; her God has told her to sell to outsiders, and if you receive medicine from the spirits, you must obey their ritual law or risk the consequences. In a similar vein, country doctors may say that their God requires them to charge for medicine. Note how this neatly reverses the usual argument that ritual laws prohibit people from selling medicine, especially to non-Kedjom. Some lay Kedjom are not troubled by this apparent circumlocution. Though it implies commerce, it is acceptable because the prices come from a God. Once fixed, however, a price cannot be changed unless the God dictates this in a new dream. Of course, some Kedjom suspect this price setting by the Gods as disin-genuous. They point to one highly commercial doctor whose practice has fallen virtually to nothing in Kedjom Keku. His therapies are worthless, they say, because he charges for medicine that he originally received freely in dreams.

Blurring the line between *tangɔ* and commerce occurs in other ways for Kedjom healers. Some say they never leave the *fon*-dom to practice therapeutically except 'by order', that is, people living outside request their services. Importantly, such clients are often said to be Kedjom; they may live outside but remain part of the *fon*-dom. This accentuates a similarity to the old compound medicine houses that always had social ties with patients, treating them at the request of the family head in his compound. By invoking this comparison, healers subtly blunt criticism that they engage in business.

Some country doctors may not charge, or ask very little for their services – avoiding charges of commercialism – yet they have consultation hours only on market day. For one healer this makes it easier for clients to buy the fowl and palm oil ritually necessary for the therapy. Intentional or not, however, it gives him access to a wider clientele; more people are in the village on market days, with more time to consult. Still other healers may increase their prices over time, but only in ritual increments. In any case, ritually set prices are common: one healer asks 1010 CFA for protection medicine, while another charges in multiples of seven: e.g., 70 CFA, 700 CFA, or 7000 CFA.[22]

As noted above, country doctors also selectively reduce prices. This might be for family members or in-laws, but also for poor or young clients. Other healers may allow poor patients to work off their debt via farm labour. Giving labour for medicine also keeps it closer to the ritual sphere. Bride-service provided by sons-in-law was far more central to marriage in the past than today. And, labour was only exchanged for cooked food or seeds, never money.[23] Other healers make it clear that their patients may 'dash' them with presents. To avoid giving gifts, of course, is considered impolite. But there may be a magical dimension as well: if patients do not give, they may feel that a successful therapeutic outcome will not last. Hence, there can be a sense of obligation that blurs easy distinction between paying a price and giving a gift.

In spite of these creative responses, the new 'traditional doctors' *have* been deeply influenced by the market. Consider one healer's comments on charging patients, a man who had recently received his medicine in dreams. It is better, he said, not to 'price man over high'. If you charge 100,000 francs (US $200, an enormous amount), 'people go deny, i [they] go come out', they will refuse to pay, and will leave. But if you ask patients to pay only 5000, then people 'go flup [full up, be plentiful] for compound'. One can see that this is an astute analysis about how low prices and high volume is a better market strategy if healers wish to earn more.

The sceptical Kedjom response to commercial medicine

How do potential clients view such bold or veiled commercialism? Some are cynical and rarely go to country doctors. Already in 1989, a good friend remarked with ironic but telling humour that at the present rate of expansion 'we *all* go be doctors'. A second woman friend 'fears' going to healers because there are 'too many' and they 'ask for goats' (that is, they are expensive), two signs that country doctors are motivated only by economic gain and do not possess genuine medicinal abilities. As she no longer knows whom to trust, she self-treats or goes to healers who treat only one or two ailments. These latter practitioners almost always ask little in compensation, and are considered less commercial; hence, they come in for less suspicion.

Other clients, of course, accept the legitimacy of the new doctors and their identity as a seller of medicine to anyone with the money to pay; and they respond by comparative shopping for the best healer, whether a Kedjom healer or an outsider. They may be sceptical, but they do not opt out of the market. Instead, they test the healer or diviner. Young men, especially, claim to bring fictitious complaints to assess the practitioner's response. Clients routinely consult multiple healers or diviners in real cases as well. By triangulating, families believe that they receive a more truthful answer. A young man noted that one should never agree immediately with an '*ngambe* man' or diviner; always say 'no', 'to push him', to see 'if he is really the correct man', if he really knows his '*ngambe*', that is, is his identity as a diviner genuine.[24]

When diviners or healers involve the spiritual world with market exchange, the Kedjom offer only limited or ambivalent approval. A number of healers, thus, have appropriated Gods, who once protected all the Kedjom, as their own private mentors. Some Kedjom accept this privatisation and commercialism, at least conditionally, while others worry it may affect Kedjom welfare. A similar split in opinion involves healers who receive medicine through apprenticeship or inheritance. For many people, these healers must charge patients the same price asked by their own teachers.[25] A daughter inherited medicine from her father to treat a childhood illness. As his medicinal heir (something new in Kedjom for a woman), she asks the same price as her father. We can see from this example that monetarising gift exchange does not mean that it is subject to market rules of supply and demand.

In spite of misgivings in the abstract, clients may still go to healers who raise prices. Kedjom are pragmatic: if healers treat complaints successfully they retain patients; if they fail to treat other ailments, then word may spread that the healer has over-reached. Either they are claiming to treat an ailment for which they have no medicine, or they have medicine but have ruined it by charging too much. Many Kedjom avoid going to one local healer because of his repute for 'liking money' and itinerating. Yet, other people grudgingly admit that for psychiatric disorders he is still effective.

Any healer who itinerates also risks suspicion and the spoiling of their identity. In 1998 four healers routinely sold medicine outside Kedjom Keku, and each incurred distrust. Even other country doctors may criticise what they consider the most commercial of all medical practices. They say bluntly that to 'walka for medicine i no fine', to itinerate selling medicine is not right. 'Walka' in Pidgin connotes irresponsibility, a rootless anonymity epitomised by harlotry. Prostitutes are women who 'walka up and down'. Medicine, too, that is not grounded in place, that is not Kedjom-specific, raises cautionary flags. Cut adrift from the ethical sphere of local ties – epitomised by gift exchange and the idealised, harmonious world of the ancestors – medicine 'for money' seems oxymoronic, and courts disaster.

The most radical case of distrust in Kedjom Keku (and the most controversial medical identity) is when outsiders sell medicine at the local eight-day market. Hausa and other venders buy daily licenses, issued by the provincial government, to sell 'country medicine'. Others lade their stalls or head pans with patent medicines, numerous balms or skin lotions. Although medicine sellers are rife, apocryphal warnings are equally legion: as strangers who may never see one again, they can make all sorts of fallacious claims, duping clients of their money. Or, worse, their medicine may be pernicious, adulterated or even poisonous. It is this impersonal exchange, solely for monetary gain, that is anathema to the medicinal sphere.

In spite of this, some clients have begun to go outside Kedjom Keku for healers and diviners. They seek better value for money and/or reject Kedjom healers as corrupt or too familiar with local problems to give accurate answers. Yet, going to a presumably neutral person elsewhere has its drawbacks: patients or their families may not know who is reliable. It may take time and cost more, given transportation and other expenses. These days, however, one need not travel to reach 'foreign' healers. Even in villages, practitioners from outside may set up shop for a few weeks, months, or years. As I noted above, an Oku man recently spent several months in Kedjom Keku at the invitation of a local healer, and with the approval of the *fon*.

Many practitioners are aware that their clients are sceptical, that they seek treatment less often now, or that they are more painstaking in selecting a healer. Healers may speak candidly about how patients are looking for lower prices and a good bedside manner. A young country doctor claims that this consumer pressure has led him to keep down his fees, and to take care in how he treats patients and their families. Yet, in the end, the moral critique of healers – about the legitimacy and veracity of their identity – may lead to a trajectory of boom and bust in their practices. It is no accident that two healers who are widely seen as the most commercial, have virtually lost their local practice. Some Kedjom say they will not go to these healers because they have ruined their medicinal power by charging fees or charging too much. Others say that when healers raise their prices, people who are jealous of their wealth may bewitch them or send bad medicines to harm the medicine. In either case, the medicine is worthless, so why go?

When a healer's local repute collapses, he or she may turn more to a non-Kedjom clientele. This means itinerating outside or receiving foreign clients at home. Either way, the Kedjom object more to healers who charge or increase fees for fellow Kedjom than for others. If healers raise prices for villagers it may spoil their medicine *and* harm the practitioners. If they do so with strangers, it affects only the client, not the healer, a version of *caveat emptor* and a moral distinction that Kedjom find less objectionable.

Establishing identity in an 'economic crisis'

In Kedjom, doubts about medical identity have sharpened since 1985 when the price of Cameroonian coffee and cocoa plummeted on the world market. Farmers earned little or nothing for their coffee for over a decade. Complicated by mismanagement, corruption, and austerity measures imposed by international lending agencies, the economic crisis has affected urban middle classes as well as rural people. The civil service, once one of the largest in sub-Saharan Africa, has been slashed by at least a third, while salaries are down 50–66 percent. In the 1990s, especially, employees might not see their pay-cheque for months, or retirees were forced to pay bribes to receive a percentage of their pensions. As a result, there was a reverse migration with urbanites coming home to farm. Kedjom elites bought large tracks of land for commercial tree crops; others raised cattle, manufactured soap, opened schools or invested in banks or other businesses. Non-elites went into truck gardening, sold used clothes, and so on.

As I have said elsewhere, an extraordinary range of creative responses occurred to make a living, including a proliferation of country doctors (Maynard 2004). While the number of healers continues to rise, clients have not kept pace; with so little cash, markets saturate quickly. Healers recognise that patients have become fewer since the crisis. Many practitioners give three reasons for this: in Pidgin they say 'Gods don high', 'doctors don high' and 'poor don come'. That is, more doctors are present, in part, because more Gods are bringing medicine to people in dreams. All of this is coupled to economic hard times when few people have money to spare. Add to this the fact that more young men are also buying medicinal knowledge from other healers to set up practices, and it is easy to see that supply exceeds demand.

Given these pressures, it is not surprising for clients to look carefully at the medical identity of healers, both their reputation for honesty and their ability to heal (related propositions to be sure). As I have said, people are astute in assessing country doctors. A young teacher once observed that as a patient you 'must play a game'. Healers may pretend 'they are serious', but they are not really 'seeing beyond' with mystical clarity into your health. Or, they may have only partial insight; they may see you are not sick, but they do not realise you are testing them. As a result, the teacher said, they give you 'lie, lie medicine, just to get money'. And, someone with fake medicine is by definition a charlatan, without a legitimate medical identity at all.

Such charges pre-date the economic crisis. One country doctor claims that some healers in the 1950s played 'tricks' to 'make business'. He says he was 'like an assistant' to the first commercial healer in Kedjom. Doctors would make a pact together. They would take phonograph needles, mix them with medicine and carry them about. Spying a potential customer, a healer would 'push [a magic] button, shoot man' in the back with a needle; crying with pain the person ran to a healer. The latter would remove the needle, receive his fee and then split it surreptitiously with his colleagues with whom he made the pact.

This apocryphal story of healers joining together is reminiscent of the many accounts of secret witch societies in pursuit of wealth or status.[26] The moral is: healing and business do not mix. This doctor refuses to distinguish ethically between such 'tricks' and 'tricks of the trade'. A doctor who deceives people to take their money, and one who uses a ruse like sleight-of-hand to increase the confidence of the patient, are equally pernicious in his eyes. Only genuine medicinal power is acceptable.

Conclusions

The commercial, universal, and anonymous nature of the new 'traditional medicine' can make it deeply suspect. Unlike the old medicine houses that pre-date European rule, the new healers treat Kedjom and non-Kedjom alike. The new medicine also incurs suspicion because of its reigning principle of payment, charging what the market will bear. To accuse healers of asking market prices is tantamount to saying that their medicine is worthless, despoiled by greed. By turning medicine into a commodity sold for private gain – and especially to outsiders – healers remove it from the arena of *tangə* and ritual exchange that circumscribe the Kedjom community.

Note the paradox in the medical identity of the new doctors: they are both too private and too public. They practice individually and make a personal profit from medicinal knowledge meant to benefit all the Kedjom. Yet, they also are too open to selling medicine to anyone, even outsiders. Divorced from ritual exchange, medicine becomes an impersonal commodity emptied of the local social ties essential to gifts. To be sure, both gifts and the market require sociality. But where the ideology of the gift requires ongoing, closely woven ties with other Kedjom, the market may be short-term and anonymous, with few or any obligations, and implies trafficking with anyone.

Where there was always tension between the market and the gift, the former is now in ascendance. Nowhere is the potential collapse of the sacred into the commercial more evident than when some healers privatise the Gods, re-fashioning the public sacra of Kedjom Keku to authenticate their personal medical practices. The old water spirits standing at the borders of the *fon*-dom are becoming the patrons of individual practitioners. By turning public Kedjom spirits into private benefactors, country doctors risk illegitimacy, spoiling the identity claims of the doctor. Taken to a logical conclusion, commercial medicine is not medicine at all, but pure hucksterism.[27]

Grassfields healers may be called, and call themselves, 'traditional doctors'. Yet, lay people may view the medical identity of such healers as anything but traditional. Nor may they call them doctors. As they depart from the old ritual ties of *tangə*, healers may be accused of having only 'lie, lie medicine'. More fundamental still, abandoning tradition may jeopardise the welfare of the *fon*-dom, just like the old ambivalence about the market. Of course, social intercourse with strangers (especially for personal gain) may be seen as a viable alternative in these hard economic times. But medicine is too powerful to be reduced solely to profit. Even good medicine, Kedjom say, should not be treated so lightly as to be taken from one *fon*-dom to another. Of course, as I have said, people in the Grassfields are practical: many still go to healers and diviners, and not all practitioners are equally accused of commercialism or of sapping their medicinal power for the sake of profit. Yet, for both healers and their *fon*-doms, making money from medicine may be risky business indeed.

Acknowledgements

This chapter addresses the Kedjom of the Republic of Cameroon. Although I discuss some of these data elsewhere (Maynard 2004), I include additional information here and analyse it from a different perspective, the social (re)production of medical identity. Ethnographic work in Cameroon has been conducted over six extended stays between 1981 and 2003, for a total period exceeding 26 months. I wish to thank the Wenner-Gren Foundation for Anthropological Research, which funded research in the summer of 1981 and again in 1989–90. Denison University, through the kind auspices of a Robert C. Good Fellowship, as well the Denison University Research Foundation and Professional Development Grants-in-Aid, funded the remainder of my research trips. I am equally grateful to the Department of Anthropology at the University of Buea for a professional affiliation while working in Cameroon. Much of this essay was written while I was an Academic Visitor at the Institute of Social and Cultural Anthropology, University of Oxford; let me thank especially Professors David Parkin and Marcus Banks, Head and Acting Head respectively of the Institute, for extending such a gracious welcome during my stay. The chapter began life at the kind invitation of Shirley Ardener, and her co-conveners Elisabeth Hsu and Ian Fowler, to participate in the seminar series 'Medical Identity' at the Institute during Hilary term of 2003. I am indebted, as always, to Susan Diduk for her close and perceptive reading of my work.

Notes

1. Although often translated as 'chief,' the *fon* (*tifon*, pl.) in Grassfields societies is more than merely a political figure. Jean-Pierre Warnier (1975) and Michael Rowlands (1987: 56) recognise his political and economic roles, but emphasise his crucial position as a mediator between the *fon*-dom and the Godly and ancestral world. Along with several priestly and medicinal societies, it was and is the *fon* who is emblematic of and responsible for the well-being of the *fon*-dom, whether health, prosperity, fertility, and good fortune generally, indeed, assuring its political sovereignty.
2. As a mandated trust territory (1914–61) Cameroon was under the auspices of the League of Nations and later the United Nations. The Anglophone area, in what is now the North

West and South West Provinces, was administered from Lagos, but received treatment somewhat different from colonies like Nigeria.

3. *Nyngong* is generally translated in Kedjom Keku as 'God.' References to local 'Gods' are also legion in both Pidgin and Standard English in Cameroon. As with Grassfields *fon-doms*, Gods are hierarchical, some concerned with the well-being of the entire society, while others are devoted to the welfare of localised lineages (or now geographical areas). Most are associated with lakes, springs or pools, especially at waterfalls (though others are said to dwell at unusual trees or stones), and are referred to on occasion as 'water spirits' (or, in Pidgin, 'mommy water'). To avoid confusion, and to repeat local parlance, I use the term 'God' to refer to all *ve nyngong* (cf. Maynard 2004).

4. As we will see, witchcraft is associated especially with strangers, that is, members of other ethnic groups. Travelling outside the village was and remains potentially perilous; whether the Kedjom go out for school, business, or simply to visit someone, they often use a variety of protective medicines, sewn into their clothes, strung around their neck, or even 'injected' (nicked with a razor blade) and rubbed into their bodies.

5. For a detailed discussion of precolonial and indigenous medicine for the Kedjom, and in the Grassfields generally, see Maynard 2004.

6. Some medicine in the precolonial era was not practised in groups, though this was the least important and most concerned with individual maladies. Individuals, like Pa discussed above, might inherit or receive such medicine from parents or relatives. Interestingly enough, this was one of the few instances where women could engage as well as men in healing. Mothers, for example, often knew remedies for common childhood complaints, such as diarrhoea, fever, or skin problems.

7. Although they practise alone or with apprentices, many Kedjom doctors have at least some ties with the local branch of the Cameroon Association of Traditional Doctors or similar groups. Similar efforts to organise healers began much earlier in colonial West Africa. By the late 1920s in Lagos, 'native doctors' were reported to form a group, in part to exclude rural healers, who were migrating to the city, whom they regarded as 'quacks' (Anonymous 1930: 17).

8. Hierarchy in the Grassfields is based on multiple principles. Although rank (achieved primarily through ritual exchange and *tangǝ*, discussed below) was crucial in the precolonial era, class has come rapidly to the fore, especially since the 1970s. Yet, gender and age also remain fundamental markers of inequality (Diduk 1987).

9. I first heard the term 'moral polity' in a conversation with Eric Worby at the Satherthwaite Colloquium on African Religion in 1997. Its use here, however, is entirely my own responsibility; for a detailed discussion see Maynard 2004: 312–15.

10. Let me note in passing a book edited by I. William Zartman 2000, *Traditional Cures for Modern Conflicts: African Conflict 'Medicine'* (Boulder, CO). Zartman suggests that, as with a good deal of indigenous medicine, precolonial strategies for diplomacy and conflict resolution in sub-Saharan Africa may be far more effective than we might think. Zartman, unfortunately, uses local medicine here merely as a metaphor. He might well have argued, however, that a great deal of indigenous medicine – like that of the Kedjom – was bound up *literally* with matters of diplomacy, conflict resolution, and the promotion of group sovereignty and welfare.

11. See Pool's discussion (1994: 159f.) of 'witch markets' for the Wimbum. Though he does not emphasise the link between witchery and business transactions, he describes how witches exchange items like food, sickness or money for a victim's life.

12. Europeans can now *tangɔ̀*, that is, give the requisite gifts to join such houses, as well as *kwyfon* and the senior priesthood and medicine societies in the palace. Still, this represents only limited access. As a 'floor member' of three groups, I have received little knowledge of specific medicinal ingredients for fear of dissipating their power.

13. Cameroonian Christians and some theologians often claim that Grassfields societies believed in one 'High God' prior to the colonial era. Local 'Gods' are said to exist, but these are manifestations of a single Godhead responsible for all creation. Still, Elias Kifon Bongmba (1995: 37f.) makes a reasoned case that the early missions imposed a 'High God' concept on Grassfields cosmologies. In support of this, few older Kedjom men and women refer to Mbe as a universal deity. Instead, they usually say Mbe created the Kedjom, while other *fon*-doms possess 'their own Mbe'. Just as Mbe made and traveled with the Kedjom, other groups travelled with their creator Gods.

14. Tellingly, the Gods (*ve nyngong*) do not protect all Kedjom. The ethnic group split into two villages, Kedjom Keku and Kedjom Ketinguh, over a dispute to the *fon*-ship in about 1860. The *ve nyngong* of Kedjom Keku protect only Kedjom Keku while Kedjom Ketinguh has its own *ve nyngong*.

15. An exception proving the rule is the early use of Hausa medicine in the Grassfields (Evans 1927: 17); that is, Hausa amulets and other medicine, brought in by outsiders, seem to have been bought and sold at market. Still, Warnier (1975: 331–2) argues for Mankon that, '[s]uccessful and dedicated medicine men sometimes had a huge clientele, coming from distant chiefdoms to consult them. They would maintain large compounds in which patients would be housed for days or weeks'. In contrast, I find no evidence of individual Kedjom 'medicine men' in the nineteenth century. Nor did healers receive strangers from 'distant chiefdoms'. 'Foreign' medicine was not allowed in Kedjom nor sought outside, for fear it would do harm. It may be that the extensive involvement of Mankon in widespread trading networks led to a different medicinal history.

16. As I suggested in note 10, ritual exchange occurred between *fon*-doms, often to end disputes or to maintain good relations. A *fon* might give a woman in marriage to another *fon* to strengthen the sense of obligation between allies. Drinking from one pot or sharing food carried a similar moral weight. Blood pacts, whether with a *fon* or a foreign trading partner, also brought erstwhile strangers and enemies under the aegis of quasi-kinship (Chilver 1966: 10). Thus, the *Fon* of Bali-Nyonga, Galaga I, asked the German explorer Dr Zintgraff to enter into a blood pact. By mixing their blood, Galega sought to ensure German support, in return promising to provide soldiers and workers (Chilver 1966: 6; Keller 1969: 26). In Kedjom, blood pacts between *fon*s could signal the end of inter-ethnic disputes (Hawkesworth 1926: para. 224). Rites also occurred when a *fon*-dom sued for peace, acknowledging its subordinate status to another *fon*-dom. This usually meant giving a leopard as an annual tribute to the dominant *fon*, though it might also entail demands for crops and other goods. The *fon* also held a royal prerogative over any python or elephant killed by groups under his control. To not give such game to the *fon* was tantamount to declaring political independence (Geary 1992: 230–1).

17. This is essentially the same as the Kom phrase, *itang iyuo*: '*Itang* … is a noun which means the act or process of counting. *Iyuo* means rank or status. … *Itang Iyuo* is the act of fulfilling certain demands of the people by going through a process [of giving] fees in cash and in kind in order to merit recognition and dignity …' (Kfutua 1994: 1–2).

18. This moral discourse distinguishing economic and ritual exchange is not unique to the Grassfields. Buying and selling, or profit taking, often connote selfishness or conduct detrimental to the group (e.g., Taylor 1992; Hutchinson 1996). *Apropos* of this, the case

studies in Parry and Bloch (1989: 2) reveal 'a strikingly similar concern [in many societies] with the relationship between a cycle of short-term exchange which is the legitimate domain of individual – often acquisitive – activity, and a cycle of long-term exchanges concerned with the reproduction of the social and cosmic order …'.

19. In the case of slavery, commerce occurred in spite of its moral disrepute but with circumspection. Marriage, too, like *tangɔ*, ought never be glossed as 'buying' a woman. Coincidentally, in the nineteenth century, bride-service was far more important than bride-wealth. In addition to labour, marriage required elaborate gifts: sons-in-law had to supply their wife's parents for some years with food, firewood, locally produced iron shovels, umbrellas, and so on. Granted, cowries and other forms of money were used as bride-wealth, but in Kedjom, prestigious crops like maize might be given instead of money for a new wife (S. Diduk, personal communication). Even with the monetarisation of marriage, beginning in the 1940s, it is impolite to speak of 'buying' a wife as though she were a slave or an object for sale.

20. Not all *fon*-doms banned the sale of subsistence food. In Bafut, food was sold at market by the 1930s (Rev. A. Suh, personal communication). Warnier (1975: 301) also notes that some *fon*-doms traded at least some subsistence crops in the precolonial era, including beans, maize, yams and groundnuts.

21. Fixed terms for ritual exchange may be honoured only in the breach. Involvement in global markets increased sharply in the Grassfields after the Second World War. With increased employment and cash crops like coffee, some ritual exchanges have succumbed to inflationary pressure. Bride-wealth, especially, has gone up dramatically. Many Kedjom argue that the influx of wealth, after the return of local soldiers by 1945, spurred inflation in the cost of marriage. In spite of such pressure, other forms of *tangɔ* have proved more stable. Both the items and amounts given to enter *kwyfon* or palace and compound medicinal houses have remained essentially the same for several generations. Nor do they always entail high payments. What was once a major expense – a goat, fowls, food, and corn beer – may be less onerous by current standards.

22. In the latter case, the healer did not escape censure for his growing commercialism.

23. Unlike money, which can be given quickly, labour requires a longer, mutual exchange. Even bride-service is never one-sided. The husband working on his father-in-law's farms, or hauling firewood for his wife's mother, always brings something home with him. So, too, patients working in the farms of their country doctor come to enjoy a closer, ongoing tie with the healer and his or her family.

24. Clients are not obligated to pursue treatment with a healer who asks an exorbitant price. Another friend noted that if a healer asks the proverbial goat, people should not dither waiting to amass sufficient resources: instead, they should begin treatment immediately with another doctor who charges less. Again, we see here the influence of the market. The medicinal relationship no longer assumes long-term social ties, deep mutual knowledge, or trust. *Caveat emptor* has come to medicine. Yet, as with any market transaction, the buyer need feel no compunction about seeking the best deal. Nevertheless, while the Kedjom have clearly grown more wary of diviners and the new healers, going to several practitioners might have occurred in the precolonial era as well. Seeing what multiple diviners have to say about a vexing problem, for example, rather than relying only on one, was the prudent thing to do.

25. Some Kedjom say that country doctors who purchase medicinal knowledge may charge what they like. However, if they in turn sell their therapies to others, they must charge only what they originally paid.

26. The idea that witches join houses called *munyongo* or *kupé* is relatively new for the Kedjom, and derives from the Bakweri and other coastal groups. These witches sell a person's life or limbs in exchange for getting ahead financially or in their careers.

27. Let me repeat that lay clients are far more likely to charge healers with quackery, of lacking medicinal power, than with being medicinally powerful purveyors of 'bad medicine' (translated at times as 'sorcery'). The closest one comes to the latter accusation is when country doctors (almost always thought to be 'boys', avaricious and without scruples) are said to sell medicine to young women wanting to abort unwanted children, a heinous act in a society that honours fertility.

References

Anonymous. 1930. *Annual Report on the Southern Provinces of Nigeria for 1929*. Lagos: Government Printer

Bongmba, E.K. 1995. 'African Witchcraft and Otherness'. Unpublished Ph.D. Dissertation, Iliff School of Theology, University of Denver.

Chilver, E.M. 1966. *Zintgraff's Explorations in Bamenda; Adamawa and the Benue Lands 1889–1892*. E.W. Ardener (ed.). Buea: Ministry of Primary Education and Social Welfare and West Cameroon Antiquities Commission.

Diduk, S. 1987. 'Paradox of Secrets: Power and Ideology in Kedjom Society'. Unpublished Ph.D. Dissertation, Indiana University, Bloomington.

Diduk, S. and K. Maynard. 2001. 'A Woman's Pillow and the Political Economy of Kedjom Family Life'. In *Family and Religion in Diverse Societies*. S.K. Haweknecht and J.G. Pankhurst, Eds. pp. 324–343. Oxford: Oxford University Press.

Evans, G.V. 1927. 'Bikom Assessment Report'. Typescript, Bamenda. Buea Archives Office File No. Ad/2.

Geary, C.M. 1992. 'Elephants, Ivory, and Chiefs; the Elephant and the Arts of the Cameroon Grassfields'. In *Elephant: the Animal and its Ivory in African Culture*. D.H. Ross (ed.). Los Angeles: University of California Press.

Goffman, I. 1963. *Stigma: Notes on the Management of Spoiled Identity*. Englewood Cliffs, NJ: Prentice Hall.

Hawkesworth, E.G. 1926. 'An Assessment Report on the Bafut Area of the Bamenda Division, Cameroons Province'. Typescript, Bamenda. Buea Archives File no. Ab/2.

Hutchinson, S. 1996. *Nuer Dilemmas: Coping with Money, War, and the State*. Berkeley: University of California Press

Keller, W. 1969. *The History of the Presbyterian Church in West Cameroon*. Buea: Radio and Literature Department of the Presbyterian Church in West Cameroon.

Kfutua, B.E. 1994. '"Itang Iyuo" as a Means of Achieving Public Recognition and Dignity in the Kom Traditional Society (An Ethical Evaluation)'. Unpublished Dissertation (Second Degree). Bambui: St Thomas Aguinas' Major Seminary.

Lantum, D.N. 1985. *Traditional Medicine-Men of Cameroon: The Case of Bui Division*. Traditional Medicine Census Report Series No. 1. Public Health Unit, University Centre for Health Sciences (UCHS/CUSS). Yaounde: University of Yaounde.

Last, M. and G.L. Chavunduka (eds). 1986. *The Professionalisation of African Medicine*. International African Seminars N.S., no. 1. Manchester: Manchester University Press in association with the International African Institute.

Maynard, K. 2002. 'European Preoccupations and Indigenous Culture in Cameroon: British Rule and the Transformation of Kedjom Medicine'. *Canadian Journal of African Studies* 30(1): 79–117.

———— 2004. *Making Kedjom Medicine: A History of Public Health and Well-Being in Cameroon*. Westport, CT: Praeger.

Ngalame, N. 1998. 'Traditional Medicine Practitioners Seek Government's Assistance to Weed out Quacks'. *The Herald Observer* 628 (3–5 July): 7.

Ngwa, F. 1998. '"Aids Is Being Cured in Africa" – Dr. Fai Fominyen'. *The Post* 3 (20 April): 8.

Perry, J. and M. Bloch. 1989. 'Introduction: Money and the Morality of Exchange'. In *Money and the Morality of Exchange*, J. Parry and M. Bloch (eds). Cambridge: Cambridge University Press.

Pool, R. 1994. *Dialogue and the Interpretation of Illness; Conversations in a Cameroon Village*. Oxford: Berg.

Rowlands, M. 1987. 'Power and Moral Order in Precolonial West-Central Africa'. In *Specialization, Exchange and Complex Societies*. E.M. Brumfiel and T.K. Earle (eds). New York: Cambridge University Press.

Taylor, C.C. 1992. *Milk, Honey, and Money: Changing Concepts in Rwandan Healing*. Washington, DC: Smithsonian Press.

Scott, J. 1978. *The Moral Economy of the Peasant, Rebellion and Subsistence in Southeast Asia*. New Haven: Yale University Press.

Shiyntum, B.W. 1998. 'Bui Tradi-practitioners Warned Against Destructive Medicine'. *The Herald* 611 (25–26 May): 5.

Warnier, J.-P. 1975. 'Pre-Colonial Mankon: The Development of a Cameroon Chiefdom in its Regional Setting'. Unpublished Dissertation, University of Pennsylvania, Philadelphia.

Zartman, W.I. (ed.) 2000. *Traditional Cures for Modern Conflicts: African Conflict 'Medicine'*. Boulder, CO: Lynne Rienner.

4

SEXUAL ORIENTATION AND GENDER IDENTITY AMONG ZULU DIVINERS

Gina Buijs

Introduction

The practice of divination is a worldwide phenomenon, wellknown from classical Greece and Rome, Japan, China, India, the Middle East and the Americas. Until relatively recently, the study of the arts of divination has tended to be included in lengthier discussions by anthropologists on religious systems, witchcraft or spirit possession. But the diviner and the process of divination are more than mere adjuncts of spiritual knowledge: as Peek notes, 'a divination system is often the primary institutional means of articulating the epistemology of a people' (1991: 2). Peek observes that, much as the classroom and the courtroom are primary sites for the presentation of cultural truths in the United States, so the diviner is central to the expression and enactment of local cultural truths, as they are reviewed in the context of contemporary realities. Divination systems are not *reflections* of aspects of a culture; they are the *means of knowledge* that underlie and validate everything else.

Contemporary Zulu people, in both rural and urban settings in South Africa, continue to rely on divination, both as a means of explaining past events and of predicting the future, and as mediation between the living and the ancestors. The *abaphansi*, or people living below the earth, are dead lineage members who continue to constrain, not to say plague, the lives of their descendants.

In this chapter I will begin by introducing the Zulu diviner (sg. *isangoma*, pl. *izangoma*) and refer to the herbalist (sg. *inyanga*, pl. *izinyanga*) before discussing gender roles and sexuality in relation to Zulu diviners.[1] While most writers on divination among the Zulu have mentioned the feminine aspect of divination, it is only recently that researchers have suggested that the profession of diviner may provide a culturally and socially acceptable role in African societies for homosexuals or lesbians.

In using terms such as 'homosexual' and 'lesbian', I am well aware that they are, as (1993: 28) Gilbert Herdt points out, nineteenth-century constructs; likewise, recent socio-historical studies of sexuality and gender show that a one-sex paradigm composed of a canonical male with a female body inside was predominant in Western texts until relatively recently (1993: 22). Herdt notes the extraordinary influence of the hermaphrodite in Western culture and art, which demonstrates the tension between systems of sexual and/or gender classification and definitions of 'nature' and 'society'. In more recent times the importance of what Herdt refers to as sexual dimorphism, or the imperative for reproduction with two distinctive sexes, helped to impel the biomedical sexological tradition towards an essentialist legacy.

After the Second World War in the West the concept of identity emerged most strongly in contexts of new social and political formations, in popular culture and in science. Particularly in studies of national character, childrearing and personality, the notion of identity became increasingly influential for psychological, cultural and gender theorists. Brigitte Bagnol (2003: 1) notes that the gender identity of a person refers to the basic nucleus of traits and characteristics by which a person recognises him or herself, and by which he or she relates to others. This description does not preclude the fact that some people may experience multiple or contradictory identities; the construction of a gender identity is a lifelong process of socialisation in which physical, anatomical (or hormonal) characteristics play a part but are not sufficient in themselves. Gender identities are influenced but not determined by social expectations, and certainly gendered behaviours and attitudes are equally affected by these expectations.

Bagnol makes the point that most social roles associated with gender have little to do with sexuality or sexual expression. Certainly, in the West gender roles are apparent most often in terms of social roles adopted in the community. Yet, in African societies, to coin a generalisation, gender and sexuality form a closer bond, as my material indicates.

Izangoma and *izinyanga,* diviners and herbalists

The distinction between a diviner (*isangoma*) and a herbalist (*inyanga)* is much like Evans-Pritchard's (1937) famous distinction for the Azande between witchcraft and sorcery, which has been found to be largely irrelevant in many other African societies. Most Zulu diviners today also act as herbalists; they prepare and prescribe their own medications for cases where such treatment is needed. Zulu diviners agree that in the past a diviner did not prescribe medication; instead, after conducting a divination session to ascertain the cause of the misfortune or illness, they would direct the client to an appropriate herbalist for treatment. The major distinction between the diviner and herbalist was in the calling or revelation of the vocation. Most herbalists were and are male, and he usually served an apprenticeship with his father or other family member. His trade was learnt; in contrast, no diviner will admit to human aid in acquiring his or her esoteric knowledge. All are adamant that their divining powers have come to them unsought from particular ancestors who were diviners themselves.

The process by which diviners become aware that an ancestor spirit wishes them to undergo training as a diviner is generally a long and tortuous one. Most Zulu diviners indicate that they felt a general weakness in their bodies. Pain in the shoulderblades and back is a generally recognised sign of possession by an ancestor spirit. Afflicted persons begin to lose interest in food and may lose weight as a result; or they may refuse to eat certain foods. An emaciated look was formerly regarded as a sure sign of spirit possession (but today is more likely to be seen as an indication that the person is suffering from AIDS). Visits to hospitals and Western doctors fail to bring about any improvement in the patient's condition, which may deteriorate and include signs of extreme impatience and irritability with others. The afflicted may wander aimlessly in the countryside, talking to themselves. Worried family members and friends will consult established diviners who advise that the patient be taken for diagnosis to a diviner of repute. Sometimes the possessed persons may say they have walked a long distance, 100 km or more, not knowing where they are going and arriving, seemingly by chance, at the home of the diviner, who will diagnose their affliction as ancestral possession and with whom they will train (Ngubane 2003: 18).

Once the affliction has been diagnosed as ancestral possession, patients are told that they must sacrifice a goat. This sacrifice signifies that the man or woman has accepted the 'call' of the ancestor and is now an apprentice or *ithwasa*. While apprenticeship is a lengthy and expensive process that may last as long as four years, it is also a time of sexual abstinence. The pupil diviner or *ithwasa* is regarded as a child during this time, not an adult, and must remain pure and refrain from all contact with sexually active men and women. Naturally, this prohibition is unwelcome to the partners of most initiates and many men forbid their wives to accept the ancestral call to become a diviner (Berglund 1976: 139). 'Barring' the ancestor spirit in this way – because of the restriction on sexuality – is considered dangerous. It may result in the patient's illness becoming more prolonged and severe, possibly resulting in death.

When the call has been accepted, the *ithwasa* or apprentice diviner leaves his or her home and lives with the tutor diviner for the period of training. As well as receiving tuition in divination techniques – specifically in methods of contacting the ancestors through dreams and by shaking or quivering (*ubikizela*) – the apprentice must also perform often onerous domestic chores for the tutor, such as fetching water, or working in the fields. The purpose of much of the instruction is to persuade the ancestral spirit responsible for the call to take up residence in or on the initiate and enable her to divine.

Gender division among diviners

Anthropologists have emphasised the female dominance of divination practices among the Nguni peoples (of whom the Zulu are part) (Bryant 1917; Hammond-Tooke 1955, 1962; Lee 1969; Ngubane 1977). The reasons given for female dominance are either psychological or sociological. Hammond-Tooke suggests that the majority of diviners among the Bhaca (near neighbours of the Zulu to the south) are women, 'probably due to the fact that the profession necessitates a highly emotional, semi-hysterical state'. He goes on to say that 'a strong-minded and intellectual woman may manipulate an opportunity to raise herself above the common level of wife and motherhood and become a respected, wealthy and influential member of society' (1962: 245). Harriet Ngubane, herself a Zulu anthropologist, maintains that divination is 'a woman's thing' and writes:

> if a man gets possessed, he becomes a transvestite as he is playing the role of daughter rather than that of a son. For the special and very close contact with the spirits is reserved in this society for women only – women who are thought of as marginal and can thus fulfill the important social role of forming a bridge between the two worlds. (1977: 142)

Hammond-Tooke (1962: 246) maintained that, 'those [diviners] who did appear psychopathic to me were the men. I knew three or four and all were distinctly neurotic and moody. One or two appeared homosexual'. However, he does not provide evidence for why they appeared homosexual, other than, 'their speech was rapid and excited, interposed with a nervous giggle'.

Writing of his research in the KwaNgwanase area of northern Kwa-Zulu Natal, bordering on Mozambique, in the late 1990s, Chang notes that 'there is no doubt that women's subjective social position in Zulu society causes tension and stress that could well find cultural expression in spirit possession', but he maintains, 'it is hazardous to stereotype divination as a "woman's thing"', for it excludes historical and regional variations' (2002: 69). Referring to Shaw (1985, 1991), he observes that there are many African societies in which the female role is restricted and minimised. In some of these societies divinership is exclusively taken by senior males or there is a gendered division of types of divinership. James Stuart, describing Zulu military conscription in the time of King Shaka (early nineteenth century), notes: 'The whole manhood of the country was liable for service. In practice, however, a few exceptions were allowed – among them diviners and those physically and mentally unfit' (1913: 68).

In his own survey of diviners in the KwaNgwanase area, Chang found almost as many male as female diviners (11 to 15). What is more interesting than the distribution of the sexes is Chang's observation (2002: 70) that:

> 'it is undeniable that the status of diviners is symbolically feminized. Diviners are regarded as 'wives' or 'daughters' to their divining spirits. Once the novice completes

training and becomes a fully fledged diviner, (s)he achieves an independent identity (that of *mungoma*). Among diviners in KwaNgwanase, novices are regarded as daughters and tutor diviners are addressed as *baba* (father), even when female. The gendering of the diviner's role is taken further in this area because the novice 'daughter' can in turn become a 'father' and usually does once he or she enrolls initiates as 'daughters' at a later stage of life.

Chang concurs with Peek's assertion (1991a: 196) that a diviner accommodates the features of 'both sexes' in one individual, and that this androgynous state symbolises the ambiguous state of a diviner who does not belong to either gender but synthesises and transcends both. Chang suggests that the symbolic attire of diviners is further indication of this androgynous state: male diviners may dress in female attire and female diviners may carry spears (*umkhonto*), a knobkerrie (*iwisa*) and shields, all symbolic markers of maleness.

Rodney Needham remarks that one of the most widespread means of transformation is inversion or reversal, and that a particularly common example of this is to be found in the institution of transvestism: 'it is common that a medium between this and the spiritual world, though a man, wears women's dress, adopts a woman's demeanour, or in many other respects assumes symbolically a status that is feminine' (1979: 39). For Needham, inversion is frequently used to mark a boundary between peoples, between categories of persons, between life and death. In an earlier account of role reversal among the Nyoro, Needham quotes from the missionary Gorja – who published his account of the Nyoro in 1920 – to note that an initiate into the Cwezi cult,

> is given to believe that he must demonstrate his genuine possession by the spirits by *becoming a woman.* [The novice] endures long torments while his initiators overbear him with accusations that he must be lying about his spiritual fitness since he has not changed sex. He is not thought to pass this test, for when he is admitted as an *mbandwa* the chief officiant asks him ironically whether he really imagines that a man can change into a woman. ... a woman candidate must submit to the reproach that she has not become a man (1973c: 316, emphasis added)

Needham himself makes it clear that he is not interested in any actual homosexual or lesbian behaviour in diviners, but only in symbolism and analogy. 'Liaisons are made indirectly by analogy and not by the positing of direct resemblance or equivalence or analogy' (1973a: xxix). Yet he seemingly contradicts this intention when he refers to the Ngaju of south Borneo among whom

> most religious functionaries are priestesses and religious matters are so intimately associated with the feminine that men who professionally assume such functions also assume feminine status. They wear women's clothes and dress their hair like women; they are commonly homosexual or impotent, and they even marry men. A man who has thus assumed femininity is thought to be more efficacious in the supernatural sphere than a woman (1973b: 117).

Androgyny or symbiosis of the masculine and feminine thus seems to be a widespread characteristic of a healer's identity. In southern Mozambique Brigitte Bagnol identified transvestism and homo-attraction among male diviners as a noticeable trait. A female healer from Maputo said,

> you find homosexuals mainly among healers. They pretend that they incarnate a female spirit only to justify their sexual behaviour. Myself, for example, I have a masculine spirit and I am not going around with suit, tie and hat. The spirit that took possession of me is a man but I got married and I have a normal life. (Bagnol 2003: 3)

In Gaza Province of Mozambique a male healer became famous for wearing women's clothes, earrings and on weekends or holidays he wore make-up like a woman. When he was asked why he did this, he said he felt like a woman because he incarnated a female spirit. This healer did not use his own name and preferred to be known as 'Madalena'. A man who became involved with Madalena and was abandoned by his wife as a result, complained at the local police station that the spirit of the healer seduced him. Madalena was forced to take off his clothes at the police station to prove he was not a woman. He was fined and told to stop wearing female clothes.

The forcible disrobing of Madalena is paralleled in the account of a black lesbian, Vera Vimbela, of her childhood experiences in rural South Africa.

> I shocked the whole village when I was in Standard Six[2] when a rumour spread that I had proposed love to another girl. It's true, I was madly in love with this girl … my grandparents and I were called to the village chief and his council of elders. The whole village turned up to the hearing, to insult me and make nasty comments. They assumed that I must be a *stabane*, a hermaphrodite, with both male and female genitals. I was taken to a hut where a woman forced me to undress and examined me. When I was discovered to be 'normal' the chief ordered that I be lashed. I was warned never to repeat such behaviour again. (quoted in Swarr 2003: 6)

Swarr notes that the Zulu term *stabane* is used in South African township vernacular to refer to an intersexual person. To be called *stabane* is to be seen as having a body that is not strictly male or female. In contemporary Soweto there is an assumption that those who identify as lesbian or gay may be *stabane*. For township dwellers, being *born* intersexual is unavoidable, while *choosing* same-sex attraction is a case for ostracism. Sexual attraction can be more easily understood and accepted when it has a physical basis, and pardoned when homosexuality can be explained through an intersexed body (Swarr 2003: 3).

Diviners' associations: *impande* and *isibaya*

In KwaNgwanase diviners and novices constitute a pseudo-kinship structure among themselves, called *impande*. This word literally means 'root' but also refers to a specific herb associated with being able to divine. The term implies the genealogy of a particular association of diviners or *izangoma*. One of Chang's informants, Jabulani, said that the *impande* is 'like a family tree'. The *impande* stands for the line of succession that is passed from trainer to trainee, from 'father' to 'daughter'.

Bernard, writing of her own initiation to a well-known diviner in 1997, says that the *isibaya* (similar to the *impande*) serves to denote the indigenous associations of diviner-mediums, that is, the collection of diviners to which one is connected through training (1999: 11). The line of succession is established or constructed by each living diviner by way of legitimising his or her claims to be a diviner. Thus, the *impande* has the secondary meaning of denoting an indigenous association or sodality. While it represents a line of connections stretching into the past, it also links a number of living diviners together into a kind of hierarchical structure of seniors and juniors.

Vertical connections are translated as parent-child relationships, specifically father-daughter. Lateral connections are transposed into 'sister-sister' sibling relationships, that is, daughters of the same father. Needham notes that for the Nyoro the word *mutende,* denoting handmaid and concubine, also means 'pupil of diviner' (1973: 316). The point is that these structured relationships form a body of knowledge known only to diviners.

The *impande* or *isibaya* is of crucial importance to diviners. It does not merely bestow a group identity but forms a corporate group. A corporate group is usually identified by its common estate, here a store of accumulated knowledge in which all members share equally. Between them the diviners exchange information on disease, medicine and other matters concerning divination and are unwilling to inform others outside the 'family' (Chang 2002: 74). Junior diviners, who train together, are solemnly bound by ties of cooperation and mutual support. For an important ritual such as the graduation ceremony of a fellow diviner, all 'sisters' as well as 'fathers' must be invited. Other diviners who do not belong to the sodality may be invited, but they remain observers only.

Eros and sexuality in the lives of diviners

I have devoted some time to the divining associations because they provide the arena, in some cases, for what appears to be an erotic association between 'father' and 'daughter'. That an erotic component may accompany these relationships can be seen in the account given by Penny Bernard of her apprenticeship to a diviner she called Baba in 1997. Baba first experienced the call to become a diviner when he was ten years old. He trained with different teachers over the next seven years and today claims that, because of his power and popularity, he has trained, directly and indirectly, over 4,000 *izangoma*. Baba has at any one time over 20 resident *ithwasa* or novices, and more who are employed and can only visit him for training at weekends. While Bernard writes that the novices behaved towards Baba with 'great respect', she also observed them 'flinging their arms around him in affection'. Hammond-Tooke (1962: 246) noted of his Bhaca diviners that, 'after a séance, the diviner (if a man) would sit among the young men and boys and joke and sing with them. One, in particular, was extremely popular with the children, who treated him very much as a white child would treat a favourite uncle, clinging to his hands and climbing on his knees whenever he paid a visit'.

On returning from a potentially hazardous journey to Zimbabwe to assist Bernard in 1997, 'Baba was nearly knocked to the ground by hordes of relieved novices and *izangoma* struggling to kiss and hug him'. As well as being outstanding as a singer, dancer and orator, she says that Baba, 'displays great compassion over people who are suffering severe affliction and misfortune and I have seen him draped over the afflicted in floods of tears'. However, she adds, 'his major weakness is his desire for glamour and his delight in prestige and wealth, especially at the expense of his competitors. This has the potential for his undoing as it goes against the moral ethic of the *isibaya* (*impande*) and provides a ready target for rivals who wish to discredit him' (1999: 8).

One of Baba's graduates, Sophie, who had no success in attracting clients in the two years since her graduation, and whose husband was becoming impatient for her to return the large investment he had made in her training, accused Baba of being a fake and a sorcerer. Baba had allegedly tricked people into believing he had been 'called' under the water by his ancestors who appeared in the form of a snake. Sophie said Baba actually had a snake familiar (referred to as an *inunu*, or monster). Victor Turner, writing on Ndembu divination, mentions a figurine called *Chanzang'ombi*. This is a wooden snake with a human face, which represents a sorcery-familiar called *ilomba*. *Ilomba* is believed to swallow its victims gradually, beginning from the feet and proceeding upwards. Only people who have drunk a potion called *nsompu* can see this happening. For others, the patient appears to be suffering from a protracted illness (1961: 8, 12).

An erotic dimension is added by the fact that Sophie had a number of dreams of engaging in sexual intercourse with Baba; this was explained as Baba sending his *nunu* at night to seduce women. Zanele, a fellow novice, agreed that she had similar dreams. Sophie then accused Baba of being a homosexual who was unable to have (presumably actual) intercourse with women. Baba's two children, she said, had been conceived on his behalf by his elder brother. That impotence is seen as an attribute of sorcerers can be seen from Turner's account of a medicine used by the Ndembu, made from a nerve in the root of an elephant's tusk. In ritual contexts this nerve is called *nsomu*. Turner comments that, because the nerve resembles a limp penis, it often has the meaning of masculine impotence. In divination it has the further meaning of a sorcerer. *Nsomu* is also a suitable symbol for death, as impotence is regarded as a kind of death. When an impotent man dies, a black line is drawn with charcoal from his navel downwards and over his genitals, indicating that his name, and with it certain vital elements of his personality, must never be inherited by the children of his kin. This is social death, and known sorcerers are treated in the same fashion (Turner 1961: 3). Diviners, as medical practitioners, are closely associated with sexuality, because for an African man or woman sexual dysfunction is commonly seen as illness, and sexual performance is equated with health and harmony with the natural and social world.

Despite calls for sexual and moral probity on the part of *izangoma* and their novices, jealousy abounds. Differing powers and skills of healing and competition for clients and novices provide rich potential for allegations of witchcraft against other members, or for the alleged use of *muti* (medicines) for negative and self-interested purposes. Sometimes *izangoma* may accuse herbalists (*izinyanga)* of sorcery (or vice-versa). Bernard (1999: 16) mentions a young male *ithwasa,*

> whom Baba had given preferential attention to, to the extent that it had led to a rift in a very special [her words] existing friendship Baba had with another *isangoma*. The youth was accused of being an *inyanga* who had become an *ithwasa* by trickery. He had been seen putting *muti* in his eyes, which, he confessed was to 'make himself look nice' for Baba.

Hammond-Tooke notes that 'there is often considerable rivalry between diviners and various medicines are used to attract clients. One, called *ibekamuandodwe* "to look at me alone" is a bulb which is chewed and rubbed on the hands and face.' (1962: 249). Further afield, Peter Fry writes of cult leaders in Belem, North-East Brazil, noting that a *pai de santo* is a magician-counsellor who provides explanations of and solutions to his clients' problems. A successful *pai de santo* is expected to have a large *terreiro* (cult house), many *filhos* (followers, literally children), good drummers, splendid rituals and much food and drink. Magical efficacy brings in the cash, while conspicuous consumption attracts clients who are the source of the income. Cult leaders who play a feminine role are known as *bichas*. The *bicha* role combines feminine attributes (cooking and embroidery) with interactions as males in the Brazilian 'world of men'. But Fry makes the important point that 'the cult leader who adopts the *bicha* role is not a would-be woman; he is in a category apart and can use the privileges associated with both female and male' (1986: 149)

Evidence that male diviners may be homosexual, and not merely symbolically so, as John Beattie and John Middleton aver (1969: 224), appeared in an interview I conducted with Sipho Ngcobo in southern KwaZulu-Natal in October 2002. When I met Sipho he was wearing a long wrap-around skirt with shirt, a form of garb that he said he found most comfortable. Sipho, who is 43, left school at 15 and migrated to the city where he found work first as a gardener and later as a cleaner and a cook in a working-class white suburb of Durban. Sipho was proud of his ability to cook, iron, and bake cakes, and noted that one employer had taught him to bake wedding cakes. While African men were widely employed as domestic servants in colonial times in much of Africa, this was not the case in South Africa. The 1980s were the heyday of grand apartheid and few working-class white women would have felt comfortable working alongside a heterosexual African male in their kitchen or laundry. Sipho, in contrast emphasised his good relationship with his employers and the interest they took in him.

Sipho described the call of his ancestors to become a diviner as a feeling of having a heavy load on his shoulders. He was told in a dream to consult a certain *isangoma* who lived in the nearby African township of Umlazi. When Sipho approached her to become an initiate, a chicken was killed to welcome him and Zulu beer offered to his ancestors. The particular ancestor 'calling' Sipho was his father's mother. Another informant, Bobby Madonsela, whose father was a water-diviner and his brother a diviner in Germiston, near Johannesburg, insisted that an initiate would take on the gender and sexual characteristics of the ancestor who was calling him or her to become a diviner. 'If I'm a lady', said Bobby, 'my voice changes to that of a man if my *idlozi* (ancestral spirit) was a man'. He added, 'if your *idlozi* was a prostitute you will also be a prostitute'. Bobby mentioned a female diviner living near him, a Miss Mthethwa. 'Miss Mthethwa is not married, her *idlozi* is a male. She behaves like a man. She walks like a man, she talks like a man. She has no husband or boyfriend. Her family don't mind.' Miss Mthethwa is about 37 years old and has been an *isangoma* for the past ten years. Bobby said she practises as a *sangoma* and people respect her. The remark that Miss Mthethwa practised as a *sangoma* was important because Bobby had previously said that although many women completed training as *izangoma*, few practised, because the diviners who trained them did not want them to work as diviners. Presumably this threat could not be applied easily to men or women regarded as men.

Bobby's information was corroborated by Mr Manqele, a 63-year-old diviner from the village of Sobokwe, near Richards Bay in northern Kwa Zulu-Natal. Mr Manqele said not all novice diviners take on the persona of women in their training: 'Things depend on the spirit that is possessing that person, when a man is possessed by a female spirit everything changes, the voice, the way he walks. If a woman is possessed by a male spirit even the way she walks will be like a man'. For his part, Mr Manqele said, he had been possessed by a male spirit.

While none of my informants commented on any explicit lesbian behaviour among female *sangomas*, film-makers Mpumi Njinje and Paulo Alberton interviewed three female *sangomas* in Soweto who set up partnerships which they regarded as marriage with other women. The *sangomas* in Soweto described their partnerships with the other women as a sexual, intimate and domestic life partnership, not different from a heterosexual marriage. One of the *sangomas*, Jama, was possessed by the spirit of her dead uncle who appeared to her in dreams saying that he wanted a wife. Jama's uncle never married, and that is how his niece explained his request. Jama married Tsidi, who is also a *sangoma* (Isaack and Gunkel 2003: 3).

After four months' training Sipho returned to his home village and began to practise divination and also to prescribe medicine for ailments. Sipho said he did this because his ancestors showed him in dreams where to get herbs from the mountains to use in healing. Sipho had both male and female clients. He said they mainly came to him for family problems, if they were feeling ill, for protection of the homestead against evildoers, for good luck, and to find lost items. For instance, said Sipho, if someone has lost a cow, he would be able to inform its owner of its whereabouts, *umhlalo umsebenzi:* he sees where things are.

Sipho said that when he worked in Durban he belonged to a Zionist church *Hlaba Hlangani*, where he was a healer or *umpropheti*. He no longer practises as a Zionist healer in his home village, just as an *isangoma*. Sipho's friend Nonhlanla, who acted as interpreter and at whose house the interview took place, told me privately that Sipho is no longer very successful as a diviner. She said Sipho does not have the patience to work hard at the business of divining. Sipho blamed family members for his lack of clients, saying that they are jealous of him. Nowadays he is usually asked for protection for homesteads, not much else.

Knowing that Sipho has never married, and that marriage is a cultural norm for Zulu men, I asked him if it was not a problem to live alone (i.e., to be unmarried). He said it was not a problem for him but that sometimes people in his village ask him why he lives alone. He said he asks such people why they ask him this: is his unmarried state a problem for them? He receives no reply. Knowing that *izangoma* are often feared for their supernatural powers, I asked Sipho if he thought such people might be afraid of him. He smiled and said 'perhaps'. Sipho said he liked being a diviner and did not mind dressing in female attire. In the old days, he said, male *sangomas* were not allowed to be married, but today this rule is not kept and male *sangomas* slaughter a goat to inform the ancestors that they intend to marry.

At this point his friend Nonhlanhla became anxious about my line of questioning and informed me that Sipho did have a girlfriend about ten years previously, but Sipho said firmly that he and the girl did not live together, 'we just visited one another'. Nonhlanhla may have been reluctant to concede to me, a stranger, that Sipho was homosexual, but she had done so to an anthropologist working in the village: 'He's gay, can't you see that?' The village was dominated by a Catholic mission and on Nonhlanhla's bookshelf was a well-thumbed copy of *The Thorn Birds* and a book of documents from Vatican Council II. Sipho often comes to Nonhlanhla's house for a plate of food, to help with cooking (as on the day I arrived) or just for a chat with his friend. I was told that rumour in the village has it that the village priest, the headmaster of the local school, and Sipho are all homosexuals and have sex with young boys. Rumour mongering of this type is not uncommon, although, as with Sipho, it is unlikely that the detractors will make their claims in public.

Evidence that homosexual male diviners may have sexual relations with boys also came from William Xulu, a young man from the rural and highly traditional area of Nkandla, in northern KwaZulu-Natal. William's father had five wives, 23 children and a large herd of cattle. He was an *inyanga* who specialised in curing sexually transmitted diseases but was also a migrant worker in a gold mine. William said that as a young child he got to know diviners by visiting the homestead of the local diviner family, the Sibiyas, when there was dancing and feasting. He said it was good fun to watch the dancing. Van Nieuwenhuijzen (1974: 25), writing of the Nyuswa people of the Valley of a Thousand Hills outside Durban forty years ago, noted that meetings of *izangoma* took place regularly, nearly every weekend in winter, and that one might then regularly meet *izangoma* on a Saturday on their way to a meeting accompanied by their pupils:

> 'mother' in full dress leading the way; the *amathwasa* painted with an extra fine touch of red or white following her. Such a procession always attracts much notice because it is graced with singing and the beating of drums which heralds their approach.

While today the red and white appears in cloth and beadwork, Turner remarks of the Luvale of Zambia, 'in the past, according to White, the diviner was daubed with red and white clay, wore a grass kilt and necklet, with a feathered headdress' (1961: 50).

Izangoma meetings are festive events with much singing and dancing, eating and drinking, laughter and talking. Van Nieuwenhuijzen (1974: 5) notes that

> many curious and interested people are also among the party, but their participation in the happening does not go beyond joining in the eating and drinking and accompanying the dancing by clapping their hands. Dancing itself is limited to the *izangoma* and their pupils. Consequently attention is continually focused on them. Even when they are not dancing they attract everyone's attention by their showy garments and their loud laughter and talking. It is their party, which they show beyond any doubt.

William Xulu explained that visits to the *izangoma* were part of the routine of the subsistence year. Every three months family elders would visit an *isangoma* to find out what the ancestors required from them, and also to be treated with medicines to keep the family, homestead and livestock healthy. These visits usually coincided with the changing seasons: 'when winter ends and summer begins, then they go there [to the *isangoma*]'. William said that *izangoma* who were homosexual preferred the company of young boys and encouraged boys to come and live with them. Parents would only discover that a *sangoma* had been involved in homosexual activities with their children when a dissatisfied client spoke about it. When I asked why parents would allow their children to live with men who might be homosexual, William pointed out that in an impoverished area such as Nkandla, where most people are poor, the *sangoma* or diviner is relatively wealthy. He can provide for these boys in ways that parents cannot.

William said that if there were complaints of a sexual nature against a *sangoma*, then, because the *sangoma* was a person of standing in the community, the matter would be referred to the local *induna* (headman) who would summon the *sangoma* to his traditional court. It was difficult to get evidence in such cases, as the children were unwilling to testify against the *sangoma* and the parents were afraid of what the *sangoma* might do to them if they laid charges against him. William said some of the children did complain, but mostly to their friends, as it was not customary in Zulu culture for children to mention sexual matters to parents. A herd-boy friend of William's had told him that when he was about 13 years old he had felt unwell and decided to consult a local *sangoma*. On arrival at the *sangoma*'s homestead, he was given a liquid to drink called *ndakabadela*. William said this medicine makes anyone who drinks it fall down unconscious (the traditional equivalent of rohypnol?). The herd-boy said that when he regained consciousness he realised that he had been sodomised. He asked a member of the *sangoma*'s household about the medicine and this person confirmed that it was used to render someone unconscious. The boy then decided to leave the diviner's homestead at once and return to his family. The diviner was one who divined with the assistance of whistling spirits (*abalozi*), who are traditionally believed to be extremely powerful and therefore feared (Van Nieuwenhuijzen, 1974: 26, 27).

Conclusion

The arrival of the HIV virus and the AIDS pandemic has led to a reappraisal of traditional attitudes to sex, sexuality and gender relations among many African people in southern Africa. In the early years of the pandemic, it was often maintained by Africans that AIDS was brought to Africa by white homosexuals from America. In discussions with university students on gender and sexuality, I have repeatedly heard it said that homosexuality is wrong 'because the Bible says so'. A recent article in the Johannesburg *Sunday Times* on the advantages of single-sex schooling for girls reads 'Despite her parents' concerns that single-sex schools bred lesbian girls and gay boys, Masigo had the final word' (24 November 2002).

Part of the reason for the general contempt and fear of homosexuality among Black South Africans may lie in the emphasis on heterosexual relations as conferring true humanity on a person. Absalom Vilakazi, writing, like Van Nieuwenhuijzen of the Nyuswa Zulu, noted:

> courting behaviour among traditional young men is a very important part of their education; for a young man must achieve the distinction of being an *isoka*, a Don Juan or Casanova. Socially, a girl who accepts a young man as a lover, even for a short time, boosts his ego and gives him status. The Zulu way of putting it is *umenze umuntu*, she has made a human being of him by recognizing him as an adult personality and as a man. To have a girl accept you as a lover is to get the assurance that you are a normal man. To fail to win a woman is to be a social failure. A man is considered as *isishimane* among the Zulu if he has failed to win a woman as a lover. A woman becomes *isishimane* if she does not get any suitors at all, or if she gets a suitor who follows her for a few days and then loses interest. Such a person is also treated with medicines to dispel the *isinyama* or ritual impurity. For a woman to be so unattractive and to lack admirers and suitors is to invite the cruel appellation of 'umgodo onganukwanja' meaning,

'a big bit of human excreta which is so odourless it does not even invite the sniff of a passing dog'. (1962: 51)

However, evidence for the existence and acceptance of homosexuality as an ordinary occurrence in precolonial Africa, not associated with military service as among the Azande (Evans-Pritchard 1970), comes from various sources (see Murray and Roscoe 1998), including a book by a well-known Afrikaans writer, C.Louis Leipoldt, first published in 1937.[3] Leipoldt recounted an episode where a 'native constable' told him of a man who had been repeatedly sentenced and punished for masquerading as a woman. Leipoldt comments, 'it was easy to identify him as a transvestite, a peculiar form of fetishism that needs treatment and not punishment'. He continued,

> in the tribe such abnormalities – or perversions as we call them – were not unknown. The native constable said that the 'old men' had told him when he was in puberty school that some men had a woman's feelings and that some women were capable of being 'ringed' i.e., regarded as men. There was nothing abnormal or incomprehensible about it. It was an ordinary accepted phenomenon that led to no a-social conduct, provided the 'young men' were properly instructed. I assured him that that was the way educated white men looked at these phenomena; but, he inquired, why then were so many natives prosecuted for practices that the native mind did not look upon as anti-social?

Leipoldt writes 'I confess I had no ready reply' (1980 [1937]: 250).

Marc Epprecht writes that recent denunciations of homosexuality by prominent African leaders have been interpreted by some observers as evidence of a perhaps essential homophobia in African culture. Epprecht considers that the real issue may be not the sexual choice but a lack of discretion or even brazenness in flouting patriarchal norms. Epprecht terms this fear of the public transgression of sexual norms transphobia, 'it implies a passive or de facto tolerance of discreet or secretive same-sex physical or emotional intimacy that in important ways has been an ally of gays and lesbians in the region' (2003: 1). He quotes an old female Shona herbalist who, when interviewed in 1998 by a researcher for Gays and Lesbians of Zimbabwe (GALZ), commented 'I've known that this [homosexuality] happens since I was a young girl and so I see nothing bad as long as it is done within closets'. The researcher asked what advice the old woman would give to gays and she replied, 'I would urge them to be quiet and keep their relationships a secret'. She added, 'in rural areas, where culture is deep-rooted, I think this [homosexuality] is understood, but the best way to deal with it is being quiet about it'.

Writing about *yan daudu*, or effeminate men who have sex with other men and *karuwai*, 'courtesans' in rural Hausaland, Stephen Pierce says that part of the reason why these groups are condemned is that they are open about their sexuality, whereas in much of Africa there is a cultural emphasis on the importance of secrecy. 'One does not share one's private business with outsiders: one does not talk about disputes for fear of exacerbating them. Behaviour that does not accord with respectability is therefore not nearly as bad if it is secret, or at least technically secret. *Karuwai* and *yan daudu* are at least partly condemned because they are open about what they are' (2003: 9).

Issues of sexuality have been highlighted in recent years in southern Africa. The constitution of South Africa proclaims equality of treatment of gender or sexual orientation, although a majority of the citizens of South Africa are unlikely to support this commitment, citing Christian teaching. In Johannesburg there is increasing visibility of same-sex identified *sangomas*, which Ebr-Vally *et al.* maintain is closely connected to the present democratic political dispensation: 'it would seem that the protection afforded by the constitution has in many ways influenced gay sangomas to come out.' But, they note, 'the coming out process is a carefully orchestrated one. For the gay sangoma is out to a few and very straight to many' (2003: 14).

Ebr-Vally *et al.* cite the case of Clive, a young gay *sangoma* who lives in Soweto but shares an office with a black lesbian *sangoma* in a formerly white part of the Johannesburg central business district. Clive insists on his gay identity having more prominence than his calling as a *sangoma*. The authors say 'the gay sangoma in the urban context has been demystified to the extent where it is no longer a prerequisite to hide one's gay status under a spiritual façade'.

For one *sangoma* a gay identity was a positive attraction. Oupa was an urban South African *sangoma* with many gay *sangoma* friends who knew of a documentary film about gay *sangomas* that created publicity for them. Oupa approached the film-makers in the hope of a similar film being made about him. When no such promise was made, Oupa became angry and the authors note, 'we had to deal with the fact that Oupa was fabricating a gay identity in the hope of obtaining personal gratification' (Ebr-Valley *et al.* 2003: 26).

The AIDS pandemic continues to grow, despite widespread campaigns by organisations such as LoveLife to promote 'safe sex' (see Hunter 2002). My research indicates that a career as an *isangoma* or diviner can provide a niche for a homosexual man or lesbian woman in Zulu society. The ban on marital relations for *izangoma* means that such individuals are recognised as being able to evade the responsibilities of marriage and family life in an acceptable and even respected manner. Evidence also suggests that, as with clergy or schoolteachers, those diviners who abuse their positions are mistrusted and feared.

While same-sex sexuality in many instances continues to be thought of as un-African by many, the *sangoma* is an African healer who is often regarded as the arbiter of African cultural values. In these terms, then, the gay *sangoma* may appear to be a contradiction. But a *sangoma* acting on the dictates of his or her possessing spirit is not acting out of personal desire; thus the community will not hold the *sangoma* responsible for transgressing limits and rules that are believed to maintain moral order in society.

Notes

1. This paper is based on fieldwork conducted with diviners in rural areas of KwaZulu-Natal, South Africa in the latter part of 2002. Names of diviners and identifying details have been changed to protect confidentiality. I have also consulted archival sources and unpublished material. I am grateful to Fiona Scorgie, M.W. Xulu and M. Ngubane for introducing me to several of the diviners mentioned in this chapter. I am also grateful to Anne Hutchings and James Kiernan for drawing my attention to the work of C. Louis Leipoldt and Yong Kyu Chang. Brigitte Bagnol, Marc Epprecht, Stephen Pierce, Amanda Swarr, and Rehana Ebrahim-Vally, as well as Penny Bernard have kindly given permission to me to quote from unpublished conference papers.
2. Standard Six is the last year of primary school, about 12 years old.
3. I am grateful to my colleague, Mrs Anne Hutchings, for bringing this book to my attention.

References

Bagnol, B. 2003. 'Identities and Sexual Attraction: Female Adolescent Rituals in Northern Mozambique and Healers in Southern Mozambique'. Paper delivered at the Sex and Secrecy Conference, Johannesburg, May.

Beattie, J. and J. Middleton (eds). 1969. *Spirit Mediumship and Society in Africa*. London: Routledge and Kegan Paul.

Berglund, A.-I. 1976. *Zulu Thought Patterns and Symbolism*. Cape Town: David Philip.

Bernard, P. 1999. 'Teacher, Trickster or Taxi Operator? Negotiating the Authenticity of Traditional Healers in Natal'. Paper presented to the Annual Conference of the Association for Anthropology in Southern Africa, Harare, January.

—— 2000. 'Guerisseurs traditionnels du Natal: une authenticitee negociée'. In *Dynamique religieuses en Afrique australe*. V. Faure (ed.). Paris: Editions Karthala.

Blackwood, E. (ed.). 1986. *The Many Faces of Homosexuality: Anthropological Approaches to Homosexual Behaviour*. New York: Harrington Press.

Bryant, A. 1917. 'The Zulu Cult of the Dead'. *MAN* 17: 140–5.

Chang, Y.K. 2002. 'The Business of Divining: A Study of Healing Specialists at Work in a Culturally Plural Border Community of KwaZulu-Natal'. Unpublished Ph.D. thesis, University of Natal.

Ebr-Vally, R., P. Riba and R.Morgan. 2003. 'Democracy, Sangomas and "Coming-out"'. Paper presented to the Sex and Secrecy Conference, Johannesburg, May.

Epprecht, M. 2003. 'Fear and Loathing of Homosexuality in Zimbabwe: A Social and Intellectual History, 1890–1980'. Paper presented at the Sex and Secrecy Conference, Johannesburg, May.

Evans-Pritchard, E.E. 1937. *Witchcraft, Oracles and Magic among the Azande*. Oxford: Clarendon Press.

—— 'Sexual Inversion among the Azande'. *American Anthropologist* 72: 1428–34.

Fry, P. 1986. 'Male Homosexuality and Spirit Possession in Brazil'. In Blackwood, E. (ed.), *The Many Faces of Homosexuality: Anthropological Approaches to Homosexual Behaviour*. New York: Harrington Press.

Hammond-Tooke, W.D. 1955. 'The Initiation of a Bhaca Isangoma Diviner'. *African Studies* 14: 17–21.

—— 1962. *Bhaca Society*. London: Oxford University Press.

Herdt, G. (ed.). 1993. *Third Sex, Third Gender: Beyond Sexual Dimorphism*. New York: Zone Books.

Hunter, M. 2002. 'The Materiality of Everyday Sex: Thinking Beyond "Prostitution"'. *African Studies* 6(1): 99–120.

Isaack, H. and W. Gunkel. 2003. 'Troubling Gender: Homosexuality in an African Society'. Paper presented to the Sex and Secrecy Conference, Johannesburg, May.

Lee, S.G. 1969. 'Spirit Possession Among the Zulu'. In *Spirit Mediumship and Society in Africa*. J. Beattie and J. Middleton (eds). London: Routledge and Kegan Paul.

Leipoldt, C.L. 1980 (1937). *Bushveld Doctor*. Johannesburg: Human and Rousseau.

Middleton, J. 1973. 'Dual Classification among the Lugbara of Uganda'. In R. Needham, (ed.) *Right and Left: Essays on Dual Symbolic Classification*. Chicago: University of Chicago Press.

Murray, S. and W. Roscoe. 1998. *Boy Wives and Female Husbands: Studies of African Homosexualities*. Basingstoke: Macmillan Press.

Needham, R. (ed.). 1973a. 'Introduction'. In *Right and Left: Essays on Dual Symbolic Classification*. Chicago: University of Chicago Press.

——— 1973b. 'Right and Left in Nyoro Symbolic Classification'. In *Right and Left: Essays on Dual Symbolic Classification*. Chicago: University of Chicago Press.

——— 1973c. 'The Left Hand of the Mugwe'. In *Right and Left: Essays on Dual Symbolic Classification*. Chicago: University of Chicago Press.

——— 1979. *Symbolic Classification*. Santa Monica, CA: Goodyear Publishing Company.

Ngubane, H. 1977. *Body and Mind in Zulu Medicine*. London: Academic Press.

Ngubane, M. 2003. 'The Calling, Training and Duties Assigned to the Sangoma: a Case Study of Mrs Khonzeni Ntombela and her Three Initiates'. Unpublished B.A. Honours dissertation. Department of Anthropology and Development Studies, University of Zululand.

Peek, P.M. (ed.). 1991a. 'Introduction: The Study of Divination, Present and Past'. In *African Divination Systems: Ways of Knowing*. Bloomington: Indiana University Press.

——— 1991. 'African Divination Systems: Non-Normal Modes of Cognition'. In *African Divination Systems: Ways of Knowing*. P.M. Peek (ed.). Bloomington: Indiana University Press.

Pierce, S. 2003. 'Identity, Performance and Secrecy: Gendered Life and the "Modern" in Northern Nigeria'. Paper presented to the Sex and Secrecy Conference, Johannesburg, May.

Shaw, R. 1985. 'Gender and the Structuring of Reality in Temne Divination: An Interactive Study'. *Africa* 55(1): 286–303.

——— 1991. 'Splitting Truths from Darkness: Epistemological Aspects of Temne Divination'. In *African Divination Systems: Ways of Knowing*. P.M. Peek (ed.). Bloomington: Indiana University Press.

Stuart, J. 1913. *A History of the Zulu Rebellion*. London: Macmillan Press.

Swarr, A. 2003. '"I Just Wonder What They Are Doing in the Bed": Secrecy, Sexuality and *Stabane* in Soweto'. Paper presented to the Sex and Secrecy Conference, Johannesburg, May.

Turner, V.W. 1961. *Ndembu Divination: Its Symbolism and Techniques*. Rhodes-Livingstone Papers no.31. Manchester: Manchester University Press.

Van Nieuwenhuijzen, W. 1974. *Diviners and their Ancestor Spirits* Amsterdam: Antropologisch – Sociologisch Centrum, Universiteit van Amsterdam.

Vilakazi, A. 1962. *Zulu Transformations*. Pietermaritzburg: University of Natal Press.

5

LEARNING TO BE AN ACUPUNCTURIST, AND NOT BECOMING ONE

Elisabeth Hsu

When I told my best friend Manu that I was thinking of studying social anthropology, she did not respond with enthusiasm. I asked her why. She said that anthropology is grounded on principles that are intrinsically flawed: anthropologists set out to observe human beings, just as animal behaviourists observed animals (she herself was a bat ethologist). She felt it was wrong that one human being should assert his or her superiority over the other by making the other an object of observation. A few years later, Manu died in a car accident, too early to learn from me that anthropologists themselves were debating and modifying their principal field method.[1]

From the beginning of my studies in anthropology, I did not want to engage in participant 'observation' during fieldwork, and it was only years later that I came to use the term 'participant experience' to designate the method with which I conducted it (Hsu 1999: 5). Engaging in participant experience meant to me that I should be involved in learning the skills and knowledge I intended to study to such a degree that I could perform those skills myself. I knew from the very beginning that I wanted to learn Chinese medicine, in Chinese and in China, but not to become a full-time doctor, because I knew I would never have the patience to treat patients. Rather, I wished to learn and use anthropological theory to understand better the complex edifice of Chinese medical theory. Also, I did not believe in studying texts only, and therefore chose sinology only as a tertiary study subject. It was knowledge as contained in everyday medical practice – embodied knowledge, we would say today –that, I then felt, would throw new light on how to approach and understand the 'logic' of the highly elaborate scholarly medical knowledge that Chinese medicine presents. This led me to study social anthropology as the primary study subject, and general linguistics as the secondary one.

Needless to say, some anthropologists were perplexed when they heard about my ideas, and they even doubted my motives. Was my intention to live for some time in China, or was it really to become an anthropologist, one of the professors asked when I began my studies in social anthropology at the University of Zurich in October 1985. I remember my feelings of indignation as I explained to him that if I had wanted to go to China – and I knew I wanted to go to South-West China – I could have gone there as a botanist; I was a fully trained botanist, and the flora of that region is famous for its richness and diversity.[2] No, it was that I felt that anthropological theory would provide a key for understanding Chinese medicine and its rationale.

I also knew from the very beginning that I wished to specialise in medical anthropology. The University of Zurich was one of the first universities in Europe to offer this subject from 1980 onwards. It had been during the first years of my biology studies, during our four-hour-long practicals in inorganic chemistry, that I would listen to the instructions given for an hour, rush over the street to attend a medical anthropology seminar for the next two hours, and only then return to start my chemistry experiments while the other students were finishing off. When the tutor came to my laboratory place, he regularly joked about my being slow and I was never quite sure whether he had observed my long absences or thought I was simply dim. He was good-natured though, and due to his private tutorials, I guess, I did well in exams.

Why study acupuncture?

It had taken me several years to be sure that it was medical anthropology I wanted to study. I did not dare to make the final step across the road for I felt that any hard-working person could make a contribution to the natural sciences, while anthropology seemed to me daunting. When I finally decided to enroll in anthropology it was again this lack of courage, or perhaps a certain degree of circumspection, that led me to learn acupuncture, *zhenjiu*, rather than Chinese herbal medicine, *zhongyi*, though I knew that acupuncture and Chinese herbal medicine were both sub-disciplines of Chinese medicine, *zhongyi*. My father is Chinese, and my Chinese relatives who spoke highly of Chinese medicine and its philosophy, which they considered mysterious (*aomiao*) and deep (*shen'ao*), looked doubtfully at me. To really understand Chinese medicine, one had to learn literary Chinese, and one had to know the Chinese medical drugs: the celebrated physician Li Shizhen, of the Ming dynasty, had described almost two thousand different kinds (Métailié 2001: 233). In acupuncture, by contrast, I then believed, one had to memorise only 365 acupuncture points, or *loci* – which is the standard number given in the classic of Chinese medicine, the *Yellow Emperor's Inner Canon* (*Huangdi nei jing*) – though there are more than that. It was important to me, as an anthropologist engaging in participant experience, that I learn a skill from the people I study to a level of competence that would enable me to perform the practice on my own. Only this level of competence would put me in a position to think about the medical theory in new ways. And, gaining a basic level of competence in acupuncture seemed less impossible than in Chinese herbal medicine.

There was also a certain elegance to acupuncture, I felt, because it involved minimal technology (needles) to effect potentially maximal therapeutic effects (instant recovery). It is generally known among Chinese people that Chinese herbal medicine acts slowly, while acupuncture has a history of being used for emergency cases (fieldwork 1988–9). Moreover, I knew from reading Paul Unschuld's *Medicine in China* (1980) that acupuncture was the therapy central to the formation of Chinese medical theory, and, for historical reasons, well worth studying.

I had not thought about the identity of the acupuncturist, however, and was soon to learn about it from a senior fellow at my graduate college when I continued my studies in social anthropology at the University of Cambridge in 1987. I was then applying for funding and overheard his flippant comment that I wanted to get my studies funded in the guise of anthropological fieldwork, in order to later get rich as an acupuncturist. So, becoming an acupuncturist in Britain was associated with making money. Not so in China.

The identity and social standing of acupuncturists in China

In general, Chinese herbal doctors do not take acupuncturists seriously: *literati* physicians wrote prescriptions while acupuncturists were grouped together with masseurs as hands-on therapists. For example, Christopher Cullen (1993: 110) observes for practices in Late Imperial China that: 'Starmaster Liu is a blind man who performs divination, heals sores, and carries out acupuncture and moxibustion. He makes manikins for the purpose of using sympathetic magic, and is generally presented as a low-life character'. Acupuncture, however, has not always been associated with the lowly. In Tang China (618–905), it was one of the four subjects taught at the Imperial Bureau for Medicine (*Taiyiju*), in Song China (960–1279) one of the thirteen (Zhen 1991: 175 and 207), and as already said, in Han China (206 BC–220 AD), acupuncture was the therapy around which the complexities of systemic medical reasoning evolved.

It was acupuncture, or rather, an innovation in acupuncture of the late 1950s, so-called 'acupuncture anaesthesia' (*zhenjiu mazhen*), that gave Chinese medicine its credibility as a science. From the late 1960s and early 1970s on, this innovation in acupuncture was performed in front of international guests who, from a gallery above the surgical theatre, could convince themselves of its efficacy with their own eyes (Hsu 1995, 1996a). In the West, people were full of admiration for this sort of 'acupuncture', which they might mistakenly equate with the entirety of 'Chinese medicine', unaware that acupuncture analgesia was a short-lived innovation, barely practised in the People's Republic of China (PRC) from the 1980s onwards (fieldwork 1988–9).

In spite of undeniable international recognition, Chinese herbal doctors often belittled the activities of acupuncturists, as did the practitioner-anthropologists who studied Chinese medicine (Scheid 2002; Ots 1990 likens acupuncture wards to day-centres). Yet, some senior acupuncturists in Kunming, where I conducted fieldwork, were well respected. Perhaps their respectable social standing was partly determined by their place of origin: two had emigrated from Shanghai to Kunming, from the centre to a border area. One of these two doctors practised a form of acupuncture not recorded in Traditional Chinese Medical (TCM) textbooks, having learnt it through the family (*jiachuan*); the other was an associate professor at the Yunnan TCM College, my college tutor.[3] These senior acupuncturists generally felt slighted at the common belief that acupuncture had no theory (*meiyou lilun*), and they spoke of theories and practices of acupuncture more elaborate than those of Chinese herbal medicine. Basic principles of acupuncture, outlined verbatim in the *Yellow Emperor's Inner Canon*, are increasingly delegated to the realm of tacit knowledge of the virtuous practitioner by the bedside. The acupuncture wards were usually close to the massage wards, and typically had beds in them, in contrast to the wards for internal medicine or gynaecology.

Eastern China is known to be the cradle of acupuncture, and though contemporary doctors did not cite *Su wen* 12 (Ren 1986: 39–40), its contents were well known to them: stone needles (*bian shi*) come from the East, drugs (*du yao*) come from the West, moxibustion (*jiu ruo*) comes form the North, and the nine needles (*jiu zhen*) from the South. Accordingly, patients in Yunnan, in the West of China, were known to believe in drugs and not in needles (*xin yao bu xin zhen*). Some therefore wondered why I had come to Yunnan to study acupuncture.[4] Indeed, the range of complaints which patients presented was very limited. Acupuncturists in Yunnan did not treat fevers and stomach-aches, as they apparently did in Shanghai, in Eastern China. Rather, they treated mostly what Chinese call the *bi*-pattern (*bizheng*): obstructions of the flow of *qi*, which manifests in pain in the joints and back.

Training to be an acupuncturist in China

Acupuncturists take the same basic courses as those who later become Chinese herbal doctors. They attend classes in Fundamental Theory of Traditional Chinese Medicine (*Zhongyi jichu lilun*), TCM Diagnostics (*Zhongyi zhenduan xue*), Introduction to Classical Chinese for Medics (*Yiguwen*), and others. A good acupuncturist is able to prescribe recipes, thus, students in acupuncture also attend courses in TCM Drugs (*Zhongyao xue*) and TCM Formularies (*Fangji xue*). Equally, a good Chinese herbal doctor is expected to be able to treat patients with acupuncture, and students are required to attend a course on the Study of Acupuncture and Moxibustion (*Zhenjiuxue*). This course addresses themes discussed in separate courses for acupuncturists: the Channels (*Jingluo xue*), the Loci (*Shuxue xue*), Needling and Moxibustion Techniques (*Zhenfa jiufa xue*), and Acupuncture Therapy (*Zhenjiu zhiliao xue*).[5]

The main memory I have now, fifteen years later, of these classes is the icy cold air in the classroom. We were wearing padded trousers and jackets, yet windowpanes were broken, and a constant draft caused cold feet and subdued stomach cramps. The hands were kept warm from incessant copying of the blackboard. I sat in the front rows, together with the other twelve women in class. This was necessary because doing participant experience involved absorbing what was said during the lecture, while sitting in the back rows, as I occasionally did later, yielded more ethnographic information on student interactions during class. There were several other incidents where doing participant experience was not ideal for observing people's interaction, but apart from many hours spent alone in my room memorising and actually learning the contents taught in class, doing participant experience was not much different from doing participant observation.

In this context, it needs to be said that I was greatly privileged to sit in class with other Chinese students. Foreign students of Chinese medicine in Beijing, Shanghai, Chengdu, and other cities were kept apart and segregated. I was the first foreign student at the Yunnan TCM College; in recognition of my biology degree, and as a postgraduate student (*jinxiusheng*), I was offered private tutorials by two of the best associate professors (*fujiaoshou*) at the college. However, given my aim to conduct anthropological fieldwork, I declined. A meeting was held at which between ten and twenty officials and teachers participated, and it took a couple of hours for me, then twenty-nine years old, to convince my senior hosts that the purpose of my study was to undergo the experience of being taught in class with seventeen-year-olds. As a result, the two tutors whom the administration had granted a year's leave for providing private tutorials were doomed to teach not only me, but a class of forty undergraduates.[6] They were excellent teachers; their lectures were lively and clear, and I hope these forty students duly appreciated their luck.

Students of vocational training attended clinical practicals in their third year, while those who became doctors attend in their fifth year; but I wished to attend practicals after just half a year of classroom training. Again, a large meeting with administrators and senior teachers was held, though a less important one than six months earlier. During that meeting my teachers were emphatic that TCM colleges provided systematic training, and by insisting on practical training by the bedside after barely having passed my first-term exams, I was exempting myself from this systematic learning (Hsu 1999: 188–9). One of my teachers flatly refused to take any further responsibility for my training as a practitioner. Yet I had paid special school fees, I was a foreign guest, and I had my way.

From March onwards, three times a week, I attended the acupuncture ward at the Provincial Hospital, about twenty minutes cycle ride away from the college. Two doctors were in the consultation room for acupuncture, several students, and barely any patients – only ten to twenty in a morning. Needless to say, I received minimal training in needling. The mornings were long, however. The doctors read the newspapers or occasionally a TCM journal; the students did the same, or we chatted. Once, very memorably, we formed a 'dragon': this meant that we practised the movements for doing massage on each others' backs, each student on the next student's back. This was the dragon, and as we shouted and laughed loudly, we almost forgot about the patients who had entered the ward.

One doctor was a chain-smoker, and it was on the acupuncture ward that I started to smoke on a regular basis. This was a very non-feminine activity, but one which had him occasionally take me to one side to show me some special Chinese medical marvel. This tutor at the Provincial Hospital was interested in studies on the *Book of Changes* (*Yijing*), as were several other Chinese doctors at the time, and intrigued by folk remedies: once he treated a woman's facial paralysis with a snake powder poultice.[7]

This doctor identified my main problem as being too timid. I was afraid of needling any patient and, when I did, I was clumsy. Patients all complained that my hand was too heavy (*shoufa tai zhong*). Instead of having them get a feeling of sourness (*suan*), cribbling (*ma*) or expansiveness (*zhang*) after insertion of the needle, it hurt (*tong*). My tutor identified the problem as my being foreign. One day, when an elderly woman with bound feet walked into the ward, he suggested I needle her, assuming that this woman was used to enduring pain. I was wearing a white coat and a white cap, and she had not recognised me as a foreigner, chatting to me in broad Yunnan dialect. However, the moment I stuck the needle into her ankle, she complained about pain and realised that I was foreign, shunning me on future visits.

On a later occasion, the tutor assigned another patient to me whom I could treat more than once. He was a young man who suffered from lethargy, hallucinations and delusions, and was diagnosed as 'mad' (*kuang*). He was sedated by psychopharmaca, but his mother believed acupuncture could lift his spirits. My tutor required this patient to be treated at very specific times of the day, which he calculated in accordance with the method of choosing *loci* on the basis of the terrestrial branch cycles (*ziwu liuzhu fa*),[8] and I was taught how to apply Sun Simiao's thirteen *loci* for treating ghosts (*shisan guixue*).[9] Nevertheless, after a few weeks this patient did not return to the ward.

I later worked in other wards of acupuncture and moxibustion. In fact, in the period of training between March 1988 and December 1989 (about which I have written little), I worked at five different wards. The college tutor who really cared about my training as an acupuncturist took me during her vacation as her personal student to her friends and fellow acupuncturists. One worked in a military hospital (I was smuggled in as though I were a local Chinese), the other in the Red Cross hospital. The Red Cross hospital, much in line with missionary hospitals in the nineteenth and early twentieth century, had initially performed mainly cataract operations, and continued to attract many patients with eye problems.[10] The acupuncturist in that hospital – a Western medical doctor forced to learn Chinese medicine in the 1950s – was inventive, and had developed needling techniques for treating myopia and strabismus. During the summer holidays his practice was flooded with myopic and cross-eyed children from the countryside; while staying with their relatives in the provincial capital, they came daily for treatment.

My apprehension of needling persisted, particularly as I was encouraged to needle in the vicinity of the eyes. It persisted even after attending classes on needling techniques, in my third term at the college, when students were asked to needle themselves in one of the *loci* on the arm, preferably the *quchi*. Patients continued to avoid being needled more than once by me. Incidentally, two Swiss friends came as tourists to China and visited me during that time. One of them, Sylvia, had menopausal flushes and had developed eczema: her face and body were covered with large red spots that itched terribly. My college tutor reacted with delight; at last the body of a foreigner presented itself and she grasped the opportunity to have me needle Sylvia daily. For ten days, my tutor came to my dormitory where we treated Sylvia on my bed, and she instructed me how to select and insert needles, whether and where to apply moxibustion. Sylvia patiently endured my clumsy needling. However, the effects were stunning and, for the first time in my life, I had an experience that must be crucial to the identity of any acupuncturist who can effect a patient's recovery.

First, I experienced enormous delight. My efforts had an effect, even though the improvement was only symptomatic and temporary: the eczema recurred a few weeks later when Sylvia returned to Switzerland. This joy that novices feel upon their first successful treatment should not be underestimated. De Martino (1988: 86) already points to it: 'It was in such an "access of mysterious and irrepressible joy" that Aua became a Shaman.'

I simultaneously experienced a feeling of empowerment. The improvement was so radical: barely any red spots were visible, and those still present were much smaller. In addition, Sylvia did not suffer insomnia and no longer complained of constant itching. It simply did not feel like a case of spontaneous recovery. Perhaps it was the care of my teacher and the concentration with which we attended to her body that calmed Sylvia down. Perhaps, it was the company she had, the leisure and fun she experienced during the outings we took into the nearby countryside. However, to me it felt as though I had an effect on Sylvia, a specific, intended medical effect; not a diffuse improvement of a psychological state but a bodily effect that was visible to everyone.

Third, I attributed the success of my treatment to my acupuncture and moxibustion procedures, and my belief in their effectiveness was enhanced. This belief in tools, apparatuses, or spirit guides, and expert knowledge, forms an indispensable aspect of the identity of any treatment provider, be it a shaman, a GP or an acupuncturist. It was not me, but me and my needles, or me and my knowledge, that had effected the improvement.

A further effect was that Sylvia later sewed me a beautiful silk jacket. Thus, I learnt yet another aspect of what it means to be an acupuncturist: in addition to whatever fee is required, patients do give personal gifts. Successful healing typically reinforces the bond between patient and healer.[11] This relation of newly acquired social dependency is often marked by material transactions from patient to healer that, in turn, makes the healer indebted to the patient and thereby reinforces the bond between healer and patient. In this way, healing becomes an aspect of social bonding and community-building.

The experience of emotional elation, a sense of empowerment, and trust in one's tools and techniques, may escape the participant observer, yet it is likely to transform the attitude of the researcher engaging in participant experience towards her subject of learning. Importantly, it made me appreciate the workings of the acupuncturist's body, on which I will elaborate in what follows. There is a multiplicity of views on the body in Chinese medicine, and as Judith Farquhar has argued (1994b), the acupuncturist's body comes closest to that of the anatomist. They are, however, not the same.

The reality of the acupuncturist's body

Today, plastic men and women are manufactured with proportions of a Western anatomical body, with lines and points drawn on the body surface in different colours. I bought one of these models because I thought it would be useful in helping me to memorise the *loci*. The plastic man was useful, but only to a very limited extent, for I actually observed myself making use of my own body instead, for memorising the *loci*. I pressed onto my skin, muscle and bone, and rubbed back and forth through the thickness of my clothes until I sensed (in my particular case) a certain kind of sourness, *suan*, and then I loudly pronounced the name of each of the *loci*. I had learnt doing so from my teachers and fellow students, and eventually, I could recite the *loci* in their proper sequence along a channel.

Knowledge of the location of particular *loci* certainly is embodied. When delivering treatment and selecting *loci*, acupuncturists in China tend to tap along the extremities with their fingers, and they typically tap the area around the *loci* more intensely before inserting the needle. By pressing directly onto the *loci*, without needling, one can already elicit the typical sensations of *suan, ma, zhang* in oneself or in the patient. No doubt, this enhances the certainty of the reality of *loci* to doctors and patients, students and their teachers (Sagli 2003: 215–18).

In addition to the *loci*, students had to memorise (in literary Chinese) the course of each channel. While I was determined to memorise the *loci*, their location on the body surface, and the specific functions they had for treatment, I never bothered to memorise the course of the channels. I was, however, fascinated by the contents of the textbook Jingluoxue (*The Study of the Channels and Links*; Li 1984), because it provided an annotated reprint of the Mawangdui vessel texts, juxtaposed to the corresponding text passages in the tenth chapter of the second book of the *Yellow Emperor's Inner Canon*, the Divine Pivot (*Ling shu*), followed by a translation into modern standard Chinese. The teacher herself read out the Mawangdui text passages, and explained some terms. The students were asked to read out and later recite the *Ling shu* text passages. I spent hours during fieldwork comparing the texts while at the same time, on the other side of the Pacific,

David Keegan (1988) had already translated and discussed them in the appendix to his Ph.D. thesis.[12]

There was extensive discussion about the reality of both the *loci* and channels, and I remember clearly an occasion where I discussed with young college teachers the undeniable effects of acupuncture, yet the oddly scientifically unproven reality of the channels and *loci* (see also Hsu 1996b). These young assistant teachers were very intelligent people with critical minds; they had been selected to study in Shanghai, for they were to be the first group of acupuncturists to teach the new course of acupuncture at the Yunnan TCM College. They were not naïve, yet their work experience would have them accept that the *loci* were 'real', and this is indeed what most believed.[13] Interestingly, however, they were not quite certain about the reality of the channels. They hypothesised that through medical practice the ancient Chinese doctors had discovered the *loci*, but that they then invented the channels, as mnemonic devices to string the points into a line. They said this although they knew that in the Mawangdui vessel texts the channels were mentioned but not *loci* – suggesting that the idea of channels along the extremities preceded that of *loci* as useful for therapeutic means.

I still remember very vividly how I felt mystified by the fact that scientists had not been able to prove the reality of either *loci* or channels; and I remember how, in discussion with these young teachers, I agreed that science had not *yet* proven their reality. Was I a gullible student? Was it participant experience rather than participant observation that led me to this attitude? Or is such identification with the beliefs and the knowledge of the people one works with a general experience of any anthropologist doing fieldwork?

Nine years later, in 1998, I was invited to give a seminar at the University of London during which I mentioned this incident and pondered over my credulity, unaware that I upset a fieldworker in the audience for aligning myself with the dominant biomedical viewpoint. Recently, in 2003, after inviting this same fieldworker (now a post-doctoral fellow) to give a seminar in Oxford, the two of us discussed the London seminar. The fieldworker, who was then working with homeopaths in South London, had since undergone similar transformations, and had more sympathy with my viewpoint, whereas I, in the meantime, had lost the certainty I displayed in London. She nodded. We laughed. And, thus, our understanding of the quality of knowledge that in some situations proves useful and therapeutically effective but is scientifically unproven seemed to meet. Probably, a purely detached observer cannot empathise with this quality of knowledge that the anthropologist immersed in fieldwork produces and that remains alive years later. It may be a quality of knowledge that the people one interacts with in the field may experience only to a limited extent themselves.

Glimpses into the history of the acupuncturist's body

There is more to say about the acupuncturist's body. Since the names of body parts refer to a static body architecture, with structures and spaces like those of an architectural building, it is perhaps best thought of as an architectural body rather than an anatomical one. However, the elaborate vocabulary used for describing the architectural body structures in the Mawangdui vessel texts disappears almost entirely from the writings that become prominent in later centuries and are most forcefully propounded in the *Yellow Emperor's Inner Canon*, which introduces humoral medical doctrine. This medicine of systematic correspondences between the five agents (*wu xing*), wind, fire, earth, water, and wood, emphasises constant flows and fluxes of *qi*, constant transformation, and this may explain why the static body-architectural terms of the Mawangdui vessel texts later lost their importance for doctors attentive to a body of humoral transformations. Yet the notion of the vessels or channels, *mai* or *jing*, as a principal feature of the architectural body in the Mawangdui vessel texts was never abandoned. It may have predated the Mawangdui vessel text writings.

Li Jianmin (1999) notes that certain *loci*, such as *tai yin* and *tai yang*, may have given the vessels their names. He thereby suggests that certain prominent *loci* were known through medical practice first, and that vessels transversing these *loci* were then postulated. At a later stage, further *loci* were projected onto the vessels. This would suggest that empirical observation combined with systematising efforts led to the elaborate system of *loci* and channels as they are known today. Li makes a very convincing argument. However, he cannot explain where the notion of vessels came from.

Interestingly, vessels as described in the Mawangdui vessel texts are visible on a lacquer figurine unearthed from Mianyang in Sichuan of the same period (He and Lo 1996). They are given red on black, with routes reminiscent of those outlined in the Mawangdui vessel texts, though far from identical. While participant experience had me engage in meditation as well, and I can testify to the subjectively experienced reality of one of these channels during meditation, the *du mai* (control channel), without further evidence it remains an anachronistic speculation whether this was also a lived reality of ancient Chinese who conceptualised the body with such vessels (as postulated by the above authors).

Even if one were to adopt He and Lo's suggestion that in the second century BC the channels reflected the inner experiences of one who mediates, one wonders where the idea of channels comes from. The experience that pressure on certain points of the body releases pain in others is variously reported (Melzack and Wall 1982: 238), while the idea of channels on the acupuncturist's body surface seems unique worldwide. Yet, perhaps they are not as unique as a student of Chinese studies may believe. Perhaps they may represent variations on a widespread cultural theme that there are routes of communication between body parts. Ducts and connections within the body and along its extremities have been recorded also in Africa (Janzen 1978: 159, fig. e) and, arguably, South America (Bastien 1989: 47). Contemporary Western depictions of the circulation of the nervous system can be viewed as representing a particularly refined and elaborate variation on this theme.

An ethnographer among the Sunuwar in Eastern Nepal pointed out that during a certain ancestor ritual, *chhegu*, strings are attached to the house altar; using the strings, the shaman is said to ascend to the altar located in the south-west corner of the house just below the roof, fetch the ancestors, and have them descend along these strings into rice figurines in a winnowing basket on the floor, where they are fed, interrogated and celebrated with song and dance (Egli 1999: 135, 322–9). A photographer in Thailand has captured the same theme of divine and spiritual energies emanating along such strings into the bodies of the community of believers (Ittipon Elajukanon in Promsao et al. 1996: 129). Considering that the term *qi* is sometimes used interchangeably with that of *shen* (spirits) and *shen qi* (spirit *qi*) in the *Yellow Emperor's Inner Canon* (Hsu 1999: 116–18), and that the modern conception of *qi* is that its flow is most pronounced along such strings or channels of the body, one cannot help but see a parallel between the movement of the ancestors, the Buddha's divine energies, and that of the spirit *qi* in the acupuncturist's body.

During the *chhegu* ritual, the *chara* (navel cord) strings which are each attached to a different compartment on the altar, are led over a bamboo ring that functions as a ritual bridge, *kya*, to hang down and connect to the rice figurines, *torma*, in the winnowing basket on the floor. Five or sometimes seven *chara* strings hang from the altar and they should not touch each other: four connect to each of the four small *torma*, and the one or three remaining strings attach to a large one. Not all *chara* strings form smooth, uninterrupted lines, however. Onto four of the *chara* strings the shaman binds (every 5 cm) seeds of the *totla* plant (*Oroxylum indicum*) that are round, transparent, parchment-like discs which are supposed to facilitate the descent of the ancestors. Egli (1999: 325) furthermore suggests that these *chara* strings can be likened to the Tibetan *mu*-cord along which the Tibetan kings descended from heaven, and which in mythical times remained attached to the top of the king's head or helmet. This *mu*-cord was likened variously to a wind pillar, a light or smoke pillar, or to a holy mountain. When a king died, his body would turn into light and ascend along the *mu*-cord into heaven. Because one of the kings inattentively cut through the cord, Tibetan kings now have corpses. There are ritual specialists, however, like Bon priests, who still can make use of the *mu*-cord, and it is also possible for lesser mortals to ascend along it into heaven after death, though divinatory and funeral rituals have to be performed for them (Stein 1989: 261–2).

Naturally, these ethnographic observations of practices testifying to the idea that spirits follow strings, and that strings connect the human to the ancestors or Buddha, are insufficient to explain why channels were and remain such a central feature of the acupuncturist's body. Nevertheless, they do uncover a cultural theme of modes of communication between humans and the divine that continue to be practised in the Himalaya and South-East Asia, and this communication along strings takes place primarily in moments of prayer and meditation. It remains to be seen whether further hints can be found to suggest that even in ancient times strings to the altar and channels within the body were routes of subjectively experienced communication with the divine.

And, finally, how I did not become an acupuncturist

Shortly before leaving the field, after having received training in acupuncture for one and a half years, I worked at yet another Kunming hospital with a much-respected senior acupuncturist from Shanghai who was truly impressed with this foreigner's knowledge of acupuncture. This approval of the skills I had acquired from several sources was very important to me; it boosted my confidence that I had sufficient knowledge to practice acupuncture in Britain. However, Sylvia was to remain the first and only patient I ever treated successfully with acupuncture.

It was not that I did not attempt to practise acupuncture in Britain, during the period of writing up my Ph.D. thesis. At the time, I felt that it would be a pity to lose the specific knowledge of a technique that I had acquired in China, and I thought I could enhance the practice of acupuncture in Britain with the skills I had acquired with Chinese students in the Chinese language in China. Indeed, there was no scarcity of patients wishing to be acupunctured, first of all myself.

Within days of returning to Britain, I fell down a steep and narrow staircase and injured my shoulder. My first port of call, as it would have been in China, was an acupuncturist (found through the Yellow Pages). The response I was given on the phone should have alerted me to the impending failure of my idea to treat patients in Britain. The acupuncturist said he would not usually treat such a shoulder injury, and asked instead if I had any other traumas. As I did not quite understand, he explained that the acupuncture he practised was good for treating psychosomatic problems.

This suggests that patients in Britain tend to consult acupuncturists when they suffer longstanding traumas (and not acute injuries of a limb). The acupuncturist in Britain thus tends to deal primarily with so-called psychosomatic problems, even if those present themselves somatically, in stiff shoulders or back pains. As an acupuncturist trained in Kunming, I was simply not prepared for dealing with such psychological complexities. Although most patients presented with problems I identified as a *bi*-syndrome, which I knew how to treat, there were further complications. I was professionally, and emotionally, not sufficiently prepared to deal with those.

Furthermore, my hand technique, which many Chinese had experienced as heavy, certainly did not please European sensibilities. I had been trained to stick needles deeply. Chinese acupuncturists do not approve of the superficial needling provided by Europeans, and European patients as a consequence are not used to deep needling. Thus, a colleague suffering from diarrhoea had constipation on the day after my treatment; a friend, intent on having her headache treated, sank into my sofa with an alarmingly pale face, minutes after I needled her.

Needless to say, such experiences discouraged me from pursuing a career as a part-time acupuncturist in Britain. Ultimately, there was no institutional incentive for a research student in social anthropology to work part-time as an acupuncturist. In fact, academics were suspicious of my activities as an acupuncturist, and some openly expressed doubts in my motivations as a researcher. I have since lost the little I acquired of the practical skills and of the more than 365 *loci* I had once memorised, only a few are still part of my repertoire. I say this regretfully, without regretting, however, the extra effort of having engaged in participant experience, and beginning to learn first-hand about the techniques, expert knowledge and identity of acupuncturists.

Notes

1. I am indebted to Shirley Ardener for encouraging me to write this very personal story and autobiographical piece. I would also like to thank Kent Maynard for valuable comments on an earlier draft.

2. In March 1986 I did one month exploratory fieldwork in an acupuncture ward in Chengdu. Fieldwork was carried out later in Kunming between September 1988 and December 1989. Kunming, the capital of Yunnan province, was the sister city of Zurich, which facilitated favourable study arrangements; in the late 1980, fieldwork requests from foreigners were generally met with a permanent *bu xing* ('it is not possible').

3. They were well respected but not as highly venerated as some of the famous doctors (*ming yi*) of the college, who practised Chinese herbal medicine (Zhang 1989: 151 ff.).

4. One of the reasons is given in note 2. My wish to study acupuncture, rather than Chinese herbal medicine, reinforced their view of me as a foreigner; i.e., foreigners were interested in acupuncture.

5. In Yunnan, in the late 1980s, acupuncture was taught at the vocational level, which involved three years of training. It was very popular with the young students, at a time when the option of setting up private enterprises or of going abroad seemed attractive to everyone. The very good students, however, would enroll in the regular five-year TCM course with its emphasis on herbal medicine (Hsu 1999: 145–57).

6. I had learnt Chinese in 1978–9 at the Peking Language School, and from 1982–84 I made my living by giving evening classes and private tutorials as a modern Chinese language teacher; already at the beginning of ethnographic fieldwork my language proficiency was sufficient that I did not need to have private tutorials.

7. Hospitals fall in the jurisdiction of the Ministry of Health (*Weishengbu*), while Colleges are under the Ministry of Education (*Jiaoyubu*). TCM professionals in the latter institutions were carefully chosen and consciously endorsed TCM principles and practices, in contrast to so-called 'senior doctors' (*laozhongyi*).

8. The method of *ziwu liuzhu* was developed in the Song dynasty, see Despeux (2001: 157); it was suppressed as superstitious during the Cultural Revolution (1966–76), but was revived in the late 1980s.

9. This patient is recorded to have been treated on 14, 16, 18, 21, 25, 28 March and 1, 4, 6, 11, 13, 15, 20, 22, 25 April 1989. From 28 March onwards, the thirteen *loci* for treating ghosts were regularly applied. In my notes the following fourteen are listed: *renzhong,*

shaoshang, yinbai, daling, shenmai, fengfu, jiache, chengjiang, laogong, shangxing, huiyin, quchi, jianshi, and *houxi.* For comparison, see Unschuld (1980: 42) and Sun (1993: 327); the names of the *loci* obviously differ. The patient was simultaneously given prescriptions, for instance, on 21 March: *chaihu* (Radix Bupleuri), *danggui* (Radix Angelica Sinensis), *chuanxiong* (Rhizoma Chuanxiong), *chishao* (Radix Paeonia Rubra), *shengdi* (raw Radix Rehmannnia), *jiegeng* (Radix Platycodi), *huainiuxi* (Radix Achyranthis Bidentatae), *zhiqiao* (Fructus Aurantii), *taoren* (Semen Persicae), *honghua* (Flos Carthami), *tiannanxing* (Rhizoma Arisaematis), *shichangpu* (Rhizoma Acori Tatarinowii), *chenpi* (Pericarpium Citri Reticulatae), *danshen* (Radix Salviae Miltiorrhizae), and *gancao* (Radix Glycyrrhizae).

10. Hsu (1992), who takes a meaning-centred approach to historical change, found evidence in the literature and among the professionals working in the Red Cross hospital in support of this statement, but not Bretelle-Establet (2002 and p.c.), whose approach is more quantitative. In her dossier of 2,000 archival notes, cataract operations were mentioned only twice (Fonds du Gouvernement Général de l'Indochine, dossier 32756, Hoihao 31.5.1900, and 56359, Semao, 5.7.1900).

11. I have characterised this as the last stage of the 'logic' that underlies interpersonal relations during ritual healing, where patienthood turns into friendship (Hsu 1999: 58–66).

12. For a published translation of the Mawangdui vessel texts, see Harper (1998: 192–212). For discussion of the vessel system in the *Yellow Emperor's Inner Canon*, see Unschuld (2003: 167–80). For discussion of the channels in a TCM book, see Porkert (1974: 197–346) and Sivin (1987: 249–72).

13. The eminent scholars Lu and Needham (1980) were intrigued by machines that can detect a change in electric voltage on the *loci,* which some consider scientific proof of the *loci's* reality.

References

Bastien, J.W. 1989. 'Differences between Kallawaya-Andean and Greek-European Humoral Theory'. *Social Science and Medicine* 28,(1) 45–52.

Bretelle-Establet, F. 2002. *La santé en Chine du Sud (1898–1928).* Paris: CNRS editions.

Cullen, C. 1993. 'Patients and Healers in Late Imperial China: Evidence from the *Jingpingmei*'. *History of Science* 31: 99–150.

De Martino, E. 1988. *Primitive Magic: The Psychic Powers of Shamans and Sorcerers.* Dorset: Prism Press and Lindfield: Unity Press.

Despeux, C. 2001. 'The System of the Five Circulatory Phases and the Six Seasonal

Influences (*wuyun liuqi*): A Source of Innovation in Medicine under the Song (960–1279)'. In *Innovation in Chinese Medicine.* E. Hsu (ed.). Cambridge: Cambridge University Press, 121–65.

Egli, W. M. 1999. *Bier fuer die Ahnen: Erbrecht, Tausch und Ritual bei den Sunuwar Ostnepals.* Frankfurt: IKO-Verlag für Interkulturelle Kommunikation.

Farquhar, J. 1994a. *Knowing Practice: The Clinical Encounter of Chinese Medicine.* Boulder, CO: Westview Press.

————— 1994b. 'Multiplicity, Point of View, and Responsibility in Traditional Chinese Healing'. In *Body, Subject and Power in China.* A. Zito and T.E. Barlow (eds). Chicago: University of Chicago Press, pp. 78–99.

Harper, D. 1998. *Early Chinese Medical Literature: The Mawangdui Medical Manuscripts.* London: Kegan Paul International.

He, Z.G. and Lo, V. 1996. 'The Channels: A Preliminary Examination of a Lacquered Figurine from the Western Han Period'. *Early China* 21: 81–123.

Hsu E. 1992. 'The Reception of Western Medicine in China: Examples from Yunnan'. In *Science and Empires. Boston Studies in the Philosophy of Science* 136. P. Petitjean, C. Jami and A.M. Moulin (eds). Dordrecht: Kluwer, 89–101.

——— 1995: 'The Manikin in Man: Cultural Crossing and Creativity'. In *Syncretism and the Commerce of Symbols.* G. Aijmer (ed.). Göteborg: The Institute for Advanced Studies in Social Anthropology: 156–204.

——— 1996a. 'Innovations in Acumoxa: Acupuncture Analgesia, Scalp Acupuncture and Ear Acupuncture in the PRC'. *Social Science and Medicine* 42(3): 421–30.

——— 1996b. 'Acumoxa in Yunnan: A Case Study of Standardising Chinese Medicine at a Medical College of the PRC'. *Journal on Southwest China Studies* 1: 217–48.

——— 1999. *The Transmission of Chinese Medicine.* Cambridge: Cambridge University Press.

Janzen, J.M. 1978. *The Quest for Therapy: Medical Pluralism in Lower Zaire.* Berkeley: University of California Press.

Keegan, D.J. 1988. *The 'Huang-ti Nei-Ching': The Structure of the Compilation; The Significance of the Structure.* Ph.D. thesis in History. Berkeley: University of California.

Li, D. (ed.). 1984. *Jingluoxue* (The Study of the Channels and Links). Shanghai: Shanghai kexue jishu chubanshe.

Li, J. 1999. 'Mingtang yu yinyang – yi "Wushier bingfang" "jiu qi taiyin taiyang" wei lie' (*Mingtang* and *Yinyang*: the Case of "Apply Moxa to his Taiyin and Taiyang" in the *Wushierbingfang* from Mawangdui). *Zhongyang yanjiu lishi yuyan yanjiusuo jikan* 70(1): 49–118.

Lu, G.D. and J. Needham. 1980. *Celestial Lancets: A History and Rationale of Acupuncture and Moxa.* Cambridge: Cambridge University Press.

Melzack, R. and P. Wall. 1996. *The Challenge of Pain.* Harmondsworth: Penguin.

Métailié, G. 2001. 'The *Bencao gangmu*: An Innovation in Natural History?' In *Innovation in Chinese Medicine.* E. Hsu (ed.). Cambridge: Cambridge University Press, 221–61.

Ots, T. [1987] 1990. *Medizin und Heilung in China: Annäherungen an die traditionelle chinesische Medizin.* 2nd revised edition. Berlin: Dietrich Reimer.

Porkert, P. 1974. *The Foundations of Chinese Medicine: Systems of Correspondence.* Cambridge, MA: MIT Press.

Promsao, K. et al. 1996. *Chiang Mai: Seven Hundred Years.* Thailand: Within Books and The Chiang Mai Chamber of Commerce.

Ren Yingqiu (ed.). 1986. *Huang Di neijing zhangju suoyin.* Beijing: Renmin weisheng chubanshe.

Sagli, G. 2003. *Acupuncture Recontextualized: The Reception of Chinese Medical Concepts among Practitioners of Acupuncture in Norway.* Ph.D. thesis at the Department of East European and Oriental Studies and the Department of General Practice and Community Medicine, University of Oslo.

Scheid, V. 2002. *Chinese Medicine in Contemporary China: Plurality and Synthesis.* Durham: Duke University Press.

Sivin, N. 1987. *Traditional Medicine in Contemporary China: A Partial Translation of Revised Outline of Chinese Medicine (1972) with an Introductory Study on Change in Present-day and Early Medicine.* Ann Arbor: University of Michigan, Center for Chinese Studies.

Stein R.A. [1987] 1989. *Die Kultur Tibets.* Berlin: Edition Weber.

Sun Simiao [681, facsimile of 1307] 1993. *Qianjin yifang* (Appended Prescriptions Worth a Thousand). Taibei: Ziyou chubanshe.

Unschuld, P.U. 1980. *Medizin in China: Eine Ideengeschichte.* Munich: Beck.

_____ 2003. *Huang Di nei jing su wen: Nature, Knowledge, Imagery in an Ancient Chinese Medical Text.* Berkeley: University of California Press.

Zhang Dehou. 1989. *Yunnan Zhongyi Xueyuan yuanshi.* Kunming: Yunnan keji chubanshe.

Zhen Zhiya. 1991. *Zhongguo yixueshi* (History of Medicine in China). Beijing: Renmin weisheng chubanshe.

6

NECESSARY IN-BETWEENS: AUXILIARY WORKERS IN A NURSING-HOME HIERARCHY

Janette Davies

Women and the workplace: caring in action

In what is predominantly a world of women, care assistants form the major part of the workforce within many residential nursing homes. We often see a high percentage of female employees, as well as a disproportionate number of women residents. At the time of my study in a nursing home in rural Oxfordshire, all thirty-two care assistants were women, as were five of six nurses. Temporary staff nurses were always women. Four kitchen staff were women, as were three out of four cleaners. Two women worked in the laundry and the housekeeper was a woman, while two men carried out the maintenance. The Manager, the Head of Care, and Deputy Head of Care were all female, as was the administrative clerk. All but one of the residents is registered with one GP Practice, which had three male doctors and one female.

The gendered nature of the workforce is echoed elsewhere in residential nursing homes, highlighted in studies such as Geraldine Lee-Treweek's (1997). Likewise, many residents in other forms of institutional care may also be women. In writing about people with dementia, Carole Archibald (1993) points out that there could be as few as one man to eight women in any activities group. Her observation is pertinent to this chapter when she says that, because care-givers (or, care assistants) are mainly women, 'the male perspective can be lost' (1993: 1).

Ethnicity in the nursing home under study also follows the trend of residential care in the UK, as all of the care assistants were white, female, and working class. The only male nurse was from West Africa, with the nursing home as his first and only employment in Great Britain. His wife, also from West Africa, worked as a night nurse in the home. All seventy-five residents were white British women and men from a variety of backgrounds, though predominantly working class. One man was born and brought up in Germany, but had spent his entire married life in the UK. No resident was from an ethnic minority group. Male entrepreneurs of British Asian heritage owned the nursing home itself. Near the end of the study, the minor shareholder bought out the major one, and two white British businessmen were appointed as financial and administrative consultants. The home then became the only nursing home within a larger group of hotels to be run by Asian entrepreneurs. In the light of government proposals for people to insure themselves for ageing and long-term care, Suzman and Rich (1996) highlighted the top ten public companies providing nursing-home care for elderly people. Prior to its sale, this present public company is one of the top ten companies in the country listed in the *Financial Times* (Suzman and Rich 1996).

In this chapter I consider the fact that paid carers, predominantly women, carry out much of the daily interaction with elderly residents, who also are mainly women. Paid care work might best be understood as work first and caring second, according to studies such as Lee-Treweek's (1995: 1). She and others show that, 'The construction of care including paid care is entangled with ideas of gender, informal care and family roles, rather than with work and ideas of occupational interest' (1995: 5).

As with nursing, the job of a paid carer is ambiguous. In the Oxfordshire nursing home, care assistants outnumbered nurses four to one, and performed many tasks similar to nursing duties. However, without professional training the care assistant has a different perspective, based on a model that most of the care assistants knew best: that of motherhood. They saw their job as an extension of their family role; most significantly for the resident, this model was primarily one of childcare and parenting. This is not without its problems, given the possibility of infantilisation, which Hockey and James (1993: 37) call 'the metaphoric transformation of older people into children'. Other studies (e.g., Ungerson 1986) find that motherhood is the model for many aspects of caring, seen as a 'relationship, rather than a set of skills and aptitudes' (1986: 65–6). We will see that the ability to act as a carer is 'imbued with sex-role stereotyping', in that mothering and caring have much in common (Ungerson 1986: 66).

Nevertheless, because of its ambiguous qualities, caring 'has defied definition', although it is socially understood as being associated with 'physical care and contact with the body' (Lee-Treweek 1995: 7). Lee-Treweek (p. 12) found that much of this paid care work was about 'containing upset and disorder by whatever means necessary'. In this chapter, I look at the way paid care work is carried out in the nursing home, in particular, how care assistants interact with residents, and how the work of the care assistant is transformative; it creates order out of disorder on any given day. Care-givers view this transformative element as part of their identity; indeed, I show how they see themselves to be the *instigators* of that transformation.

Caring and the care assistant

Throughout the study one could see that the quality of life for the resident was often dependent on the quality of working life of the employee. Life in a residential facility is as much about the workers as it is the resident; thus, my larger study – on which this chapter is based – shows how the quality of life for both resident and employee is inextricably linked. Understanding, and the need for sensitivity to the difficulties faced by both care assistants and residents in a nursing home, cannot be overestimated.

> At the centre are the main caregivers, nursing aides ... Nursing home life is as much a story of the workers and their worlds as it is of the residents, and it is important to be sensitive to the difficulties that workers as well as residents face ... (Foner 1994: vii)

One of the most significant issues to consider concerns that of training and acquiring of the skills necessary to do the job. Many of the care assistants whom I observed and worked with on a daily basis had never been offered formal training during their employment. Yet, it was evident that nearly all of them had an ethic of care. One could also see skills being acquired 'on the job', which were excellent for many of them, though lacking for others. Working on the premise that most women can and do care for family members, care-giving was an extension of the role these women would play in their home lives. Indeed, they highlighted this as part of their task, part of their identity as a care assistant.

Nevertheless, much of what care assistants do in their job 'is barely distinguishable from nursing care' (Shemmings 1996: 156). This is not just a case of residents 'becoming more physically dependent with staff needing physically to lift and feed them', but rather it is the increasing variety of situations that the staff now face in these workplaces (op. cit. p. 156).

> When on duty, staff are required to make constant adjustments according to the situation in which they find themselves with residents. Whilst some [residents] are extremely frail physically, others may hit staff or other residents; others may call out incessantly and seem to be quite unaware of their behaviour ... They may be unaware of why they are living in residential care. It is against this backdrop that residential workers care for vulnerable people who are dying. (Shemmings 1996: 156)

My research shows the tensions and dilemmas for care assistants encountered in their everyday work. From working with the care assistants in the home, I observed that these 'tensions and dilemmas' are heightened by their realisation that much of what their job consists of has traditionally been a 'nurse's job.' Care assistants state that they feel valued and recognised for doing a nurse's job, yet they resent the fact that their pay does not reflect their great responsibilities.

Patterns of care

From the following examples of what is involved in caring for nursing home residents, we can easily see that an ethos of care runs through the work of even the most informally trained care assistant. That ethos is integral to their identity as care workers. In the Oxfordshire nursing home, two of the women had been care assistants for over two decades within the institution. Two others had worked there for ten years. Although there were no formal positions for senior care assistants, these two older women, and others on different shifts, were seen to be 'senior' in terms of their acquired wealth of knowledge. Much 'training', therefore, was conducted during routine care of residents, as new care assistants were assigned to work alongside the 'seniors' to gain the skills necessary to complete tasks successfully.

A work break after serving breakfast – often only for a cigarette – gave a similar, more informal opportunity for the practical exchange of information. As there was no formal hand-over time from night to day staff, this informal break became especially important for exchanging information before the busy morning work got under way.

When such cooperation does not occur, it may reflect the status dilemmas of care assistants discussed above. For example, sickness often results in time off amongst the staff. Two care assistants said that they used to do the extra work of bathing, as well as the daily washing and dressing of residents, when someone was off sick, until they decided that 'enough was enough.' From then on they attended to the residents of the staff off sick, but would only bath their 'own quota': the workload would be unacceptable, they felt, and the regular care of their 'own' residents would decline. The reason for their decision was that they felt that management took them for granted, that the situation 'had gone on for too long', and more especially, that their 'own' residents would suffer. The care-giving was not what it would be when they had their normal workload; by caring for more residents than usual, less time was inevitably taken with each resident.

One senior care assistant showed much common sense in her work method: her organisation and practical sense were probably as much to do with her personality as with experience. For example, to find a solution to the problem of bathing a woman with long hair, after washing and rinsing it with the shower hose, she would tie it up on top of the woman's head so that it would not trail in the dirty bath water. She chose clothes efficiently if residents could not choose for themselves, but quickly consulted them whenever possible. All the time, she talked to patients, explaining what she was doing, constantly conducting her work in a caring manner. Then after each person was ready and seated in the lounge she made a cup of tea, which she considered an extra to her duties, as the next round of hot drinks was not served until 11 A.M. when all the 'chores' were done. This was an individual touch, but we can see the attention to detail and her practical understanding in getting the residents up for the day.

During tasks such as these we came to know each other by sharing personal histories. This particular care assistant was a family woman with well-loved grand-children of her own. As we exchanged our life experiences, especially concerning families, it was evident that within her family she was seen as a practical, caring person ready to help her children and grandchildren, and to be generally available as they live near her. There was a sense that she used this practical approach in her work situation, as well as the acquired knowledge gained from many years of experience. Whether she had joyous news, such as an addition to the family, or sad news such as the illness of her father, she shared it with colleagues and resi-dents alike, including them all vicariously in her family life.

Some of the residents, able and interested enough to have conversations with the care assistants about their family life, became involved in these discussions. They had a wealth of experience to offer from their own lives while the work was carried out. Some of the employees had very serious issues to contend with at home, for example bullying or petty theft. Care-givers brought these kinds of worries to their working situation each day, worries that make Hochschild's phrase 'the second shift', especially apt: 'In addition to the physical and emotional demands of work they had to manage household chores ... complicated by baby-sitting arrangements that wore them down' (Hochschild 1989: 107).

Likewise, there was a constant movement of care assistants, with a strong sense of loyalty to each other, to help lift residents when bathing and washing. This concurs with the findings of other studies, such as Foner's, where she says that, '[a] principle kept among themselves is that care assistants should help each other when needed with aspects of the job such as lifting. Not only employees benefit, but residents too' (Foner 1994: 129). Learning to help in this way is all part of socialisation into the informal rules of the workforce, and being unwilling to help was definitely viewed negatively by other care assistants.

As with many comparable institutions, a formal coffee break was not taken by the staff until all residents and patients were up and dressed. However, as we saw above, time was taken to stop and have a quick cup of coffee, or go outside for a cigarette, which the care assistants felt was acceptable. The managerial staff also accepted this as unofficial practice, although they emphasised that the work process should not suffer because of it. According to Foner:

> ... the bureaucratic division of labour in Weber's (1947) view constitutes, in many ways, a 'cage in which modern men and women are compelled to live'... [T]he rules and procedures that have developed to regulate care are often a 'cage' for nursing aides (Foner 1994: 53)

On being asked why all residents had to be attended to before lunch, even when care assistants were busy during times of staff shortages, the care assistants said that there was little flexibility and the home manager wanted it that way. The sen-ior care assistants did, however, on occasion bathe patients in the afternoon if they proved 'difficult' in the mornings, thus enabling their own flexibility within the organisation. The 'quick' cup of coffee and cigarette taken between attending to residents was also evidence of this type of flexibility or 'bending of the rules': care-givers see it as part of caring for themselves. The flexibility described here is sim-ilar to what Lee-Treweek calls 'resistance'. In her study on women, resistance and care, she describes the nursing auxiliaries' ambiguous relationships to authority as, 'an acceptance of one's place in and yet at other times a resistance to the hierar-chy': 'Rather than perceiving themselves as the victims of a strict routine, the aux-iliaries presented a view of themselves as the prime movers in its construction and maintenance' (Lee-Treweek 1997: 54).

Breaking minor rules is one way in which care assistants could show initiative: they would work around the routine as, for example, when they explained that they usually bathed Arthur in the quietness of the afternoons, rather than in the busy mornings. More time could be given to him then, especially encouraging him not to be aggressive and not to hit out. In this way they made the work eas-ier for themselves as well as for the resident.

However, there are ambiguities, even in the use of the term 'caring.' The posi-tion can give power over the weak and vulnerable, yet can be disempowering for the care assistant (or even for a relative who cares for a family member at home). For care assistants, the hard work is consistently described as stressful and the low pay as derisory. Within the hierarchy of the institution, care assistants are located at the lower echelons. The perceptions of the job associated with this low social status are all factors that produce powerlessness. Not having time to meet their own needs, such as a cup of coffee on a busy shift, or when there is staff shortage, can also add to feelings of frustration in the job.

But by the nature of the work of caring for the vulnerable, the care assistant can also be seen as occupying a position of power. Many of the ideas discussed here reflect Foucault's (1988) concept of power and power relations. Care-givers are at pains to point out that they are the workers at the 'grass-roots' level; one even remarked that they are 'at the coal-face' in keeping the system of care-giving going. However, they were also able to exert some power within their daily rou-tine by their use of flexibility or 'resistance.' Within Foucault's appraisal of power, the institutional resident has less control over his/her own life than the employee does:

> In the Western industrialized societies, the questions who exercises power? How? On whom? are certainly the questions that people feel most strongly about ... Who makes decisions for me? Who is preventing me from doing this and telling me to do that? Who is forcing me to live in a particular place when I work in another? Who is pro-gramming my movements and activities? How are these decisions on which my life is completely articulated taken? All these questions seem to me to be fundamental ones today. And I don't believe that this question of 'who exercises this power' can be resolved unless that other question 'how does it happen?' is resolved at the same time (Foucault 1988: 103).

We can consider this in terms of the bureaucracy that is part of the management of institutional life, and the way in which employees describe management as powerful especially in control over the use of time. Foner shows how bureaucracy often 'discourages initiative which results in lack of spontaneity;' it even has 'some negative consequences for patients ...' (Foner 1994: 54). Though, as we have seen, even where this bureaucracy discourages initiative, a number of care assistants in the present study were determined in their approach to undermine it, such as their flexibility in bathing a resident in the afternoon.

Yet, at times I observed an over-emphasis on organisation and a task-centred approach, which (along with bureaucracy) stifled the creativity of the employee. Bureaucracy becomes inevitable in nursing home organisation; Foner stresses that, '[n]ursing homes would be unthinkable without bureaucratic organisation – not just in terms of administrative efficiency and to ensure even minimal standards of care but to prevent serious patient abuse' (op. cit. p. 54). But bureaucracy creates certain problems and tensions. It emphasises strict adherence to rules and regulations, and can stifle spontaneity and impinges on the lives of the residents. It can also provide opportunity for revolt.

Managing difficult situations

One of the most difficult encounters with a resident for care assistants is a situation classed as 'challenging behaviour.' For many people, dementia may result in confusing, at times bizarre, frightening or aggressive actions. Many of the difficult situations faced by staff involved aggression, and occasionally pollution. One lunchtime, when I was working with an experienced care assistant, a resident became very disturbed. She shouted, banged the table forcibly and insisted that she had not ordered the meal of fish given to her, as earlier we heard her tell the kitchen assistant that she was 'sick of fish'. There was definite skill shown by the 'senior' care assistants in diffusing the situation by negotiating what the resident could eat. This kind of situation happened often, but the care assistants found ways of managing, not necessarily by having formal training, but by inherent skills of personality, as well as humour and experience. Care assistants negotiated regularly with the residents to calm their aggression and confusion, often the result of their deteriorating condition.

A challenging incident took place one weekend when there was a trail of faeces from the lounge to the toilet and another trail leading back to the lounge, after one male resident defecated on the carpet. Within the nursing home setting this has become the lot of the care assistants, as it is part of their workload to clean up after an incontinent resident. That day the lounge was filled with residents and visitors, and the latter were concerned that the care assistants had to clean it up, acknowledging how busy they had been that day, both with staff shortages, and with particularly sick residents requiring more care. Bodily functions, normally contained behind closed doors, had become public, making paramount a sense of urgency to create order out of disorder. In contrast to the visitors, both the residents (whose frailty intensified or dementia became more severe) and the caregivers responded with tolerance rather than irritation and anger.

Without the necessary training, such situations can create undue stress and tension for the employees in their endeavours to deal with the situation. To a certain extent care assistants have to face what Jenny Littlewood (1991: 170) calls 'care and ambiguity'. Although she is predominantly discussing the nursing profession, issues such as 'excreta and control', and acting as mediators of pollution, are as much a part of a care assistant's role as that of a nurse. Most of this mediation and negotiation takes place in the privacy of bedrooms, as noted by Geraldine Lee-Treweek. It was in the 'private' spaces of the residents' bedrooms that the containment of disruption, and the ordering of distress or aggression was carried out [and the] the product of the work [being a] clean, orderly, quiet resident' (Lee-Treweek 1997: 51, 54).

Although this kind of description seems a little cold when considering the care assistants in the Oxfordshire home, it is evident that a 'clean, orderly, quiet resident' leads to considerably less stress for both the care assistant and the resident. It is the management of 'dirt,' described by Mary Douglas (1966) as 'matter out of place', that is always evident in the busy morning routine, a routine that usually contains the 'dirt' before it enters the public domain.

The housekeeper pointed out that in the absence of a sluice it was regular practice to empty commode pots down the toilet, causing the contents to spill over the surround of the toilet and on to the floor. This is not usually cleaned immediately, as a cleaner has to be found. So when a resident went to the toilet and sat on the toilet seat, she or he came into contact with someone else's soiling. The risk of infection is obvious. But how does one clean commodes without a proper sluice? Even the wooden frames around the commode needed cleaning, where pubic hair and encrusted faeces were often observed. Care assistants described this and other aspects of their work as 'heavy', as with the typically 'heavy' situations of having to lift people. 'Heavy' was also used when describing other aspects of care in daily living, such as putting someone's clothes and shoes on, often the case with people in severe stages of dementia.

This paper highlights the daily working life of the employee. It centres on the circumstances faced in caring for frail and sick elderly women and men. This can be the overwhelming smell of a diaper full of faeces and urine, or the extreme pollution of the contents of a commode slopping onto the shoe or leg of a staff member. These are the harsh practical issues of work, as well as the stress of caring for someone in the years, days and hours before death. Of consideration here is the almost impenetrable world of a person suffering from the severe stages of dementia, and the daily endeavour to communicate verbally, or through other methods such as a touch or smile. That the job is often described as 'heavy,' and emotionally draining in no way detracts from the quality of care provided. Indeed, a genuine relationship may develop between the care assistant and resident. Celia Davies (1995: 141) states that although the term 'caring' is hard to define, it does involve 'the creation of a sustained relationship with the other'. I consider this relationship in closer detail later in the paper when I discuss extended family and networks within the home.

Poor maintenance and lack of equipment and supplies

Everyday concerns of care, as we have seen, matter greatly for the job satisfaction and identity of care assistants. In the home, when I worked with care assistants, discussion often took place concerning such questions as the state of the linen, bedding, and clothing. One assistant said that if she saw a really threadbare sheet she would put a hole in it and place it in the rubbish bin; otherwise the sheet returned again and again from the laundry to be used on a bed. She and others felt strongly that residents should not have such poor bedlinen, nor feel the uncomfortable contours of a mattress through a threadbare sheet. All care assistants mentioned that the linen and towels were thin and worn, and some of the quilts had split corners with the stuffing coming out. Many of the care assistants said that the soap and bath products were not good, in that the ingredients were harsh with overall low quality. Likewise, supplies that would make the care assistant's job much easier were not always available, such as wet-wipes for personal hygiene care of a resident. There were also occasions when the necessary incontinence pad was not available.

Replaceable parts

Given such difficulties, heated discussions might take place during breaks, sitting in the garden, describing working life. Especially mentioned was how the staff became ill under the pressure of what they perceive to be an increasing workload, saying that there was never enough time to get over sickness. A note of injustice was expressed, as staff were not paid during time off for any sickness. The male nurse on one occasion displayed deep scratch marks on his arms after attending to a woman resident. Other staff were spat at by one resident in particular. Menzies (1970: 7) pointed out that the physical illness suffered by a nurse 'is intensified by her task of meeting and dealing with psychological stress' in her work. Over thirty years later, the same can be said of care assistants.

When there was shortage of staff, particularly on a Monday morning, everyone appeared to feel the pressure instantly, including residents. Staff pointed out that management never looked into the situation of increased staff shortage following weekends, an indication to care-givers that management undervalued them. Diamond (1992: 187), in his covert study in a nursing home in the USA, shows that low-paid workers in such jobs as residential care are often seen to be easily replaceable.

In the Oxfordshire home, one care assistant left for a job at a veterinary laboratory, explaining that she would be paid more, with better conditions working with animals than with elderly residents in the home. These kinds of situations were often discussed amongst the staff, who did not exclude any resident within earshot who wished to join in, although female residents more than the men would voice opinions about shortages of staff and conditions.

Peace *et al.* (1997: 118) show that care workers are classed as manual workers: '[c]are workers for older people still fall generally in manual grades, and the care workforce is vulnerable to competition from local labour markets. Generally, pay is better in local hotels than in residential care.' There is an irony in this, considering that the main shareholder of the home under study was an hotelier. Within the nursing home as well as away from it, an oft-repeated phrase was 'you get paid more to pull a pint in a pub', than you do to look after a sick person.

Extended networks: family and home

The care assistants had built up strong networks of support and friendship amongst themselves, and many of the employees lived near each other on a large housing estate in a nearby village. Many of the parents of the care assistants were from the same towns and villages as the residents, thus establishing a common geography of place, if not identity. One of the women residents, whose mother had run a public house, was well known to a number of the care assistants whose parents were regular customers there, which increased mutual memories, becoming points of conversation. Two of the care assistants on the day shift were sisters, while their mother worked evening shifts. One of the female laundry workers had a daughter who was a full-time care assistant. During the university summer vacation a female student worked as a care assistant, her mother being deputy head of care as a nurse on the permanent staff. The mother-in-law of a part-time care assistant worked within administration, while the male day nurse was married to one of the night nurses. One of the male residents was the cook's grandfather he died in the home at the end of the study. Another resident's daughter-in-law was one of the night nurses.

Well known to many people on the local housing estate were one of the care assistants and her young family, who worked night shifts at the home. A huge sense of loss was felt in the home, and much further afield, when she unexpectedly died leaving a husband and small children, and grieving staff and residents in the home. Lee-Treweek (1997: 52) found a similar situation saying that there was '... an informal process which often led to daughters, sisters or nieces being asked to help out ... and ending up full time.'

Female residents were keen to share in these networks, and although none of the residents hailed from that housing estate, there were links. For example, a woman was admitted, aged well into her eighties, and had a loving attentive husband. He told me that one of his granddaughters was the girlfriend of the son of the hairdresser at the home. The hairdresser also resided on the local housing estate. Residents new to the home felt this kind of family network immediately and eventually became included in it. Relatives spoke of it being a good extra dimension to the life of the home. Women residents especially knew much about the care assistants' home background and often knew their children as well, who were encouraged to visit the home. In this way it was actively argued that the residential home was indeed a home away from home for the resident, as the manager maintained was their ethos.

Visitors, too, often had mutual workplaces in common, the most interesting and extensive being a former MG sports car factory. A number of male residents responded animatedly to photographs that the maintenance man brought in showing the factory before it was closed. Word of this MG involvement spread, and visitors began to make contact with the retired workers in the home when they visited. Where the women could share vicariously with the care assistant's lives and families, the men had a different biography to share, usually that of common workplace interest. This particular shared biography of the men, including the grandfather of the cook, in the history of the car factory was nostalgic and always aroused interest with other visitors. That the maintenance worker knew that the researcher enjoyed sports cars possibly added to the subject being aired.

Care as identity

In a discussion of the use and meanings of the term 'care,' Rosemary McKechnie and Tamara Kohn highlight Dalley's distinction between 'caring for' and 'caring about'. They suggest that 'caring for' means 'the work of tending to another's needs,' while 'caring about' is 'how one feels about another person' (McKechnie and Kohn 1999: 4). That many of the women cared about the residents in their charge, as well as their daily work, shows how residents were 'cared for', something highlighted in this chapter. Of course, without formal training – or, in some cases, ability – it is probable that not all assistants were able to do the job of 'caring for' residents. That an untrained agency care assistant with no experience of work in an institution did not feel the need to put toast on a plate – carrying it in her hand instead – is extreme evidence of this. A nurse who gave medication to two women sharing a room, without a word of greeting or conversation, evidently lacked interest in them as individuals, as well as in her job. Indeed, she left within six months of the researcher beginning fieldwork.

Relationship between management and care assistants

Throughout the study, and especially when I was working alongside the care assistants, they often described the relationship between management and employees as tense. In particular, the staff always interpreted the interaction of the female care assistants and nurses with the female manager as a negative encounter. For example, when visitors from the head office were present, one of the nurses was criticised when shampoo was found in a bathroom. It was seen to be a poison risk, as a person with the cognitive impairment of dementia could view it as a drink and ingest it. What the nurse objected to most was the style of criticism, and where it was done (loudly, in front of visitors and residents). Later the aggrieved nurse discussed the style of management, especially noting the lack of constructive criticism. She stressed that most of the employees felt that they were often criticised and rarely praised, even when they were doing extra work during staff shortages. She said that the style was always confrontational. As a result, she began to express a desire to look for new work, which she did, eventually moving to a hospital job.

She and some of the care assistants were expressing the feeling that they felt undervalued by management, by a manager that seemed to have no understanding of what their tasks involved. This was in stark contrast to the relationship built up between the Head of Care and staff; indeed, the Head constantly encouraged the care assistants. Two of the nurses had a similar approach when working with the care assistants. Alan Gilloran and Murna Downs say that good leadership, which they term 'encouraging and enabling', has to be seen at the level of actual care. They also recognise that senior management must plan for staff training needs, stressing the need for training to care for people with dementia (Gilloran and Downs 1997: 169). This, they say, contributes to higher levels of morale amongst staff members.

In contrast to this ideal situation, many care assistants explained how they did not see the manager as the 'right type'. They found her style confrontational and critical, and observed in particular that she did not 'listen to their point of view'. Linked with this was their astute perception that she never gave out praise, only criticism. I observed evidence of this negative style of management especially during a meeting called by the manager, and attended by the care assistants, laundry, cleaning, kitchen and maintenance staff. She began the meeting by holding up a piece of wire with dust around it and asked if anyone could suggest what it was. A number of care assistants guessed correctly that it was the wire from under the cup of a brassiere. It had become caught in the washing machine that was subsequently out of order and costly to repair. The manager asked what could be done to prevent this happening again. After suggestions, the manager said that the wires should be taken out of the bras and for staff to ask relatives to buy wireless bras. Finally, the manager allocated responsibility for this to the care assistants.

Consider their response to this suggestion, and its impact on their sense of identity and status. Care-givers told me afterwards that they felt treated like skivvies, cheap labour; there was evident disquiet but no one protested to the manager herself. There was no mention of consideration to those women who needed to wear such bras. The response of the employees was to seek me out regularly throughout the day, ask me what I thought about the meeting, and to state how unjust they felt some of the manager's views were.

The housekeeper discussed the staff meeting and noted how only she and one care assistant had made comments. Echoes of the 'muted voice' are heard here; using Shirley Ardener's notion of 'muted groups', we can underscore the mutedness within the nursing home setting, the unheard voice of women. Ardener (1975: xii) draws on Edwin Ardener's use of the dominant male group or model, describing how women in turn tend to be inarticulate, a 'muted group'. The domination of management over the care assistants effectively muted any voice that might wish to be heard. The housekeeper said that colleagues felt threatened and intimidated in meetings with the manager, given her argumentative manner, which most employees did not want to confront.

What was distressing about this management style for caregivers was how and when criticism was made. All were of the opinion that criticism was 'given in the heat of the moment', which often coincided with stressful, busy times for staff or after the death of a well-loved resident. I once observed such heat-of-the-moment criticism concerning a woman sitting in the lounge with no stockings on: her relatives visited one morning and found her bare-legged. The manager immediately found the nearest care assistant and criticised her for this in front of the visitors. The care assistant was not the woman's key worker, but she knew why the resident had no stockings: she was awaiting a dressing on a small skin nick in her shin, and the attendant explained this to the manager. She later told me that she felt most aggrieved by the manager's immediate response, without first finding the resident's key worker. For the care assistant who was criticised, the net effect was to feel a loss of control over the kind of blame attributed by the manager.

A second occasion of public criticism occurred when I was sitting with residents in the dining area where a piano was also located. I watched the manager pick up a pair of clean stockings left on the piano, and ask very loudly who had left them there. No one answered her. One of the nurses nearby told me that was the 'kind of question we can do without'. She noted how busy that morning's work had been, and how all the care assistants on that wing had washed and dressed extra people before lunch. It would have been far more sympathetic, she said, for the manager to thank everyone for doing extra work rather than make a petty comment about tidiness.

One area that the care assistants and nursing staff said management did not listen to, at 'grass roots level', concerned staff shortages, especially during shifts when one or more people were off sick. No extra pay was ever offered for carrying the extra heavy caseload when on duty. Two nurses related to me how they had counted the shifts on one particular weekend: thirteen shifts were not covered, which meant that existing staff had to take on the care of extra residents. Administrative and nursing staff knew in advance about the coming staff shortage – as these were planned holidays – but management did not call an agency for five additional care-givers until the day before the weekend.

Eventually, residents themselves began to comment more frequently about the shortage of staff, especially when it affected them, such as not being able to have a bath. Near the end of the study, one resident said that 'there was a constant feeling of shortage of staff and rush to get things done before shifts ended'. Staff leaving became a constant theme of discussions, and again there was the feeling that management did not value staff. Morale for both residents and staff members was low; one of the youngest care assistants said that what was needed was a 'mass staff walkout'. Only then, she thought, would management 'sit up and take note' of the workload, staff shortages, and stress of the job. The manager was seen to be unavailable. This young woman was upset as she felt that there was never any praise from management, only criticism, even when attending to fourteen residents in one morning. She eventually spoke out at a meeting of employees with management, but afterwards senior managers denied her an opportunity for overtime as a form of reprimand.

One of the nurses said that the style of management, which she described as being 'on the defensive', resulted in staff thinking that they could not negotiate with management about such issues as sick pay. Also, membership in a trade union had always been discouraged, so care assistants had become used to not having a forum for labour issues, such as the non-payment of sick pay. Some of them tried to explain to the manager, to no avail, that they often became sick because of working in the nursing home environment, with its difficult and taxing demands. They also felt that with few or no formal qualifications they had little choice in the wider job market, other than within residential care settings. As a result, these women felt deeply that they were 'at the mercy of the employer', especially relating to salary and working conditions.

New management

During the course of the study, I observed staff morale decline until the manager resigned. On her departure and appointment of the Head of Care to the post of manager, staff morale improved greatly. When the staff met the new managers, one care assistant, employed temporarily, acted as a spokeswoman for the staff by asking whether a pay increase would be considered. The other staff described her as 'quite brave', as few employees spoke up at meetings. She had mentioned the heavy workload of care assistants within the nursing home at a meeting for regular staff, voicing the opinion that of all the nursing homes she had worked in, this one had the heaviest workload. Two of the care assistants said they were convinced that only residents were important to the management, and not employees. Another care assistant also pointed out the poor wages. In contrast to the old regime, these complaints seemed to be noted by the new managers, as a pay increase occurred within two months of the changeover.

In the days after the meeting, different staff members told me that they now felt they could approach management with ideas, especially about repairs and much-needed supplies. For example, some staff members told the managers about the need for a ramp from the conservatory to the garden, something that had been suggested two years previously without result. The housekeeper, on being asked by management what she most wanted in her work, expressed the need for different cleaning products: the present supplies did not clean well enough, and there were more suitable products on the market. The morale of the staff began to improve as some of these suggestions were quickly implemented, especially the construction of the ramp to the garden for wheelchair access or for people using walking sticks. The difference between trying to negotiate steps with a walking stick and using a ramp was noticeable to the residents, and was said by staff to enhance the quality and pleasure of residents' lives.

For some years there had been a difference in the amount paid to care assistants on the same evening shift. Some of these hours are classed as 'unsociable', yet not all the staff received extra pay for unsociable hours under the old management. This was another discrepancy sorted out early on by new management, and did much to raise the morale of those on the evening shift. Amongst the staff, and the care assistants in particular, there was a noticeable increase in morale after meeting with new management. They had felt commonly that the confrontational management style constantly undermined their endeavours for the residents, and impeded their own practice. On negotiating with the new management, the staff commented upon the difference in style and how the new managers were prepared to listen to them as individuals as well as a group. All staff, including the kitchen and maintenance staff, hoped that this characteristic of management would last. There was an impression of openness with both staff and residents about issues concerned with the home. Most significant was the construction of the ramp from the conservatory to the garden, thereby assuring something useful and visible, and an early indication of how management would respond to the perceived needs of both staff and residents. Both groups said they felt they had been listened to, that their voices had finally been heard.

Conclusion

In looking at questions of identity in this paper I also show the interaction between care assistants or nursing staff with management, and how that constructed an identity as a menial worker. Yet with new management taking over at the end of the study we can see that it was avoidable: a different professional identity came to the fore. What emerged from the study was how the identity of the care assistant (and to a lesser extent nurses) was bound up with a grass-roots level of caring for the residents. They were seen to be the 'necessary-in-betweens'. That is, they were not at a managerial level, nor at a professional level such as nurses. Rather, they were 'manipulators' of good care, in spite of the lack of supplies, shortage of staff and high levels of criticism by management. As we saw when discussing management style, staff perceived their dealings with management, and even their treatment, as inevitable and hierarchical. Care assistants were a buffer between the hierarchy of management and the consumer, client base of the residents. In other words, they were not often listened to but often criticised, frequently in public. They felt undervalued (evident especially in poor pay and conditions), but themselves placed value on the work they carried out daily, whether for the most able or the frailest resident.

Scholars have shown that the main work of a nursing auxiliary is to create a sanitised 'lounge standard' patient, fit to be on view, as opposed to the 'bedroom state' of being 'dirty physically and often mentally disordered' (Lee Treweek 1997: 53). My research also shows that a 'lounge standard' is the result of the work that the care assistant performs in the bedrooms with the residents. However, I would also suggest, having worked alongside care assistants, that they believe this is for the good of the resident and not necessarily for the public life in the lounge. Within the kind of order that results from the routine of attending to residents in the privacy of their own bedrooms, a human dignity is conferred, so that the recipient can participate in the public area of the lounge. Within the habitual routine of the care assistant, the needs of residents were anticipated and met, at the same time that a conversion from disorder to order occurred, from a bedroom state to a publicly accepted state. I have shown how this is integral to the identity and work role of the care assistant. Even without formal training, their ability to deal with many challenging and sad situations gives them a sense of value that, even when it is undermined by management, remains evident in their approach to work and the way in which they carry it out.

The deft managing of difficult situations figured consistently throughout the study; to the staff this represented a righting of disorder to achieve the desired calm order of the nursing home. The care assistants felt that they were better able to deal with this than nurses and management, and believed that the intrinsic skills involved in the job of caring for residents contributed to the overall formation of identity in that job. Inherent within this identity is a sense of authority by virtue of the fact that they are good at a job that not many people could face doing.

References

Archibald, C. 1993. *Activities* 11. Dementia Services Development Centre, University of Stirling.

Ardener, S. 1975 (ed.). *Perceiving Women.* London: J.M. Dent & Sons Ltd.

Davies, C. 1995. *Gender and the Professional Predicament in Nursing.* Buckingham: Open University Press.

Diamond, T. 1992. *Making Gray Gold: Narratives of Nursing Home Care.* Chicago: University of Chicago Press.

Douglas, M. 1966. *Purity and Danger: An Analysis of the Concepts of Pollution and Taboo.* London: Ark Paperbacks.

Foner, N. 1994. *The Caregiving Dilemma: Work in an American Nursing Home.* Berkeley: University of California.

Foucault, M. 1988. 'On Power'. In *Michel Foucault Politics, Philosophy, Culture. Interviews and Other Writings, 1977–1984.* L.D. Kritzman (ed.), London: Routledge.

Gilloran, A. and M. Downs. 1997. 'Issues of Staffing in Therapeutic Care'. In S. Hunter (ed.), *Dementia: Challenges and New Directions*. London: Jessica Kingsley Pubs.

Hochschild, A.R. 1989. *The Second Shift: Working Parents and the Revolution at Home*. London: Piatkus.

Hockey, J.L. and A. James. 1993. *Growing Up and Growing Old: Ageing and Dependency in the Lifecourse*. London: Sage.

Lee-Treweek, G. 1995. 'Understanding Paid Care Work – Towards a New Critique'. *Manchester Sociology Occasional Papers* 43. Manchester University Press.

———— 1997. 'Women, Resistance and Care: Nursing Auxiliary Work'. *Work, Employment and Society* 11(1): 47–63.

Littlewood, J. 1991. 'Care and Ambiguity: Towards a Concept of Nursing'. In *Anthropology and Nursing*. P. Holden and J. Littlewood (eds), London: Routledge.

McKechnie, R. and T. Kohn. 1999. 'Why Do We Care Who Cares?' In *Extending the Boundaries of Care: Medical Ethics and Caring Practices*. T. Kohn and R. McKechnie (eds). Oxford: Berg.

Menzies, I.E.P. 1970. *The Functioning of Social Systems as a Defence Against Anxiety*. London: Tavistock Institute of Human Relations.

Peace, S.M., L.A. Kellaher and D.M. Willcocks. 1997. *Re-evaluating Residential Care*. Buckingham: Open University Press.

Shemmings, Y. 1996. *Death, Dying and Residential Care*. Aldershot: Avebury.

Suzman, M. and M. Rich. 1996. 'Nursing Home Operators Look for Healthier Future'. *Financial Times*, 4 May.

Ungerson, C. 1986. 'Women and Caring: Skills, Tasks and Taboos'. In *The Public and the Private*. Gamarnikov, E. D. Morgan, J. Purvis and D. Taylorson (eds). Aldershot: Gower.

7

MIDWIVES' IDENTITY IN A BRITISH HOSPITAL: THE COST OF A NORMAL BIRTH

Jenny Littlewood

Historically, European midwifery was often thought of as a wise woman's role, carried out within a community amongst neighbours and kin with ongoing social ties: the status of the woman, midwife and child were clearly understood, and the midwife was known to the woman before pregnancy, and for many years afterwards. With the gradual professionalisation of medicine, and the stratification and parcelling out of the body and its functions amongst different specialities, the midwife's contact with the woman, and her role in childbirth, have been much more narrowly defined. Midwifery identity has become increasingly neutral, both morally and socially, focusing on a smaller area legitimately dealing only with 'normal' and 'successful' birthing.

Paradoxically, the separation of women who are pregnant into sections of the maternity and hospital services – which may be categorised according to the age of the foetus as well as its medical and social status – may have the counter effect of alienating the woman from the community and the possible support she could offer others as well as receive herself. The stratification of pregnancy into 'successful slices' may also have the consequence of helping to ensure funding for the institution. However, this may add to the heavy burden on the midwife to conform to increasingly technological intervention to prevent maternal and infant mortality.

Midwives are encouraged to involve partners of the labouring women in the birth situation, in response to central government policies on shared partnerships in childbirth; likewise, this may also have the consequence of helping to relieve the staffing shortage. With increasing technology and medicalisation of the experience – leading to the division of pregnancies according to their chance of success based on foetal age – midwives must work to present the birth as a 'natural event', shared in the delivery suite by people who are often strangers to her. At the same time she may need to protect her own professional identity from harm by any failure at the delivery; paradoxically, this may serve to alienate her from colleagues, as midwifery identity is intricately bound up with the successful birth of a 'normal', healthy baby.

Hospital spaces and structures

Whilst professional groups may have had distinct origins, and guard their professional identities and expertise by rules and language, these may be gradually eroded or controlled by structural changes, by external definitions and markers that change the extent and content of their practice. This chapter considers such issues through a case study of midwives in a large teaching hospital in London. The maternity departments in the hospital serve an area of high deprivation, high population density and high reproduction rates. Public Health Statistics for 2000/2001 show that the borough population, from which pregnant women are mainly drawn, forms 6 percent of the total population of London, the second highest district for population density, and the highest on most indices of deprivation.[1] The data were collected through an eight-month research project interviewing and following midwives, other professionals and pregnant women who experienced miscarriage specifically before the twenty-fourth week of development.

In the UK, neither the law nor medicine acknowledges life before twenty-four weeks. It is only after this time that life may be thought to be sustainable, and for which a death certificate is issued. If the child has breathed, a birth certificate is also issued. Whilst it might be thought that services for a pregnancy of any duration would be housed in the maternity block, in fact this is not so. In the study hospital, the professional division of the pregnancy relates to the foetal age, the likelihood of its survival, the impact on the maternity provision for successful outcomes, and the additional impact on hospital statistics, indeed, on the future funding of the service (Littlewood 2000).

The layout of the hospital, its wards, and the duties of the professionals, indicate the hierarchical relationships, and other distinguishing features of maternity provision. The hospital has expanded from its original building in 1900 to occupy an area over three quarters of a mile square. Originally, this facility was an isolation hospital for infectious diseases, changing to general use in the 1930s, adding a purpose-built maternity block in 1970s to accommodate 2,000 births. However, in 1997, the maternity facilities were managing over 4,000 births. A completely new maternity wing is envisaged for completion in 2007. The teaching block for midwives is on the lower west side of the site, and is a single-storey, renovated building. It is located behind the waste disposal services and laundry centre, and separated from the medical teaching block that is in the inner core (fig. 7.1).

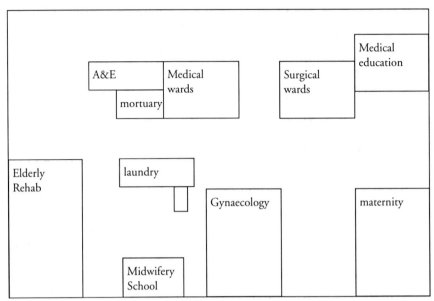

Fig 7.1 Hospital layout

The new mortuary is located in the centre of the total hospital space, beneath a small hospital chapel, and near the Accident and Emergency Department (A&E) and the administrative offices of the hospital. Nationally in the UK, midwifery and gynaecological services are housed in separate wards; in the study hospital, they occur in entirely separate buildings. Whilst doctors are both gynaecologists and obstetricians serving both disciplines, the midwives are entirely separate from gynaecological nursing: maternity services are in a new building close to medical education, while gynaecological buildings are near to buildings providing rehabilitation services for the elderly, out-patient departments for the chronic sick, and specialist services for people with cancer. Gynaecology departments provide women with specialist services for disorders and or disease of the reproductive areas of their body. However, women are directed to gynaecological services from A&E when pregnant with complications before twenty-four weeks, and where the foetus is dead or likely to die. Preferentially, the woman is sent from A&E by staff to miscarry at home. Women with pregnancies to be terminated for social reasons are also looked after on the gynaecology wards.

The maternity block is four storey high. It is staffed by a total of 156 midwives in and around the hospital, of whom twenty-six are 'bank midwives' working anywhere required if there is a shortage of midwives. Forty-three percent of the remaining 130 midwives are part-time (Hansard 2004). Of these, all the midwifery managers are white women, five out of eight Irish in origin. Of the practising midwives, 78 percent are African or African Caribbean in origin, similar to the population they serve, 65 percent of whom are African and African Caribbean.

Within the study hospital it is the clinical practitioners who wear uniforms. Uniforms may provide some distance, objectivity, respectability, recognition of authority through knowledge, and easy recognition of their peers; they also provide status and positioning within a hierarchy and divisions within midwifery. Whilst biomedicine claims to provide 'identity-free' treatment for people – treatment based on need rather than race, social class, or culture – the structure of the hospital and the uniforms provide clear divisions within the services that are equally reflected in the class, ethnic and educational divides between and within the professionals.

The spatial structuring of birth

The ground floor is for the uncomplicated deliveries serviced by a general practitioner/community unit where women come in for a few hours only. They have their babies under the care of their own doctor, or midwife who is linked to that doctor (general practitioner). Should complications arise, they can be transferred upwards. The midwives in the GP/community unit have uniforms, and work in teams of four with three shifts. They may work in a very confined space with many tiny cubicles (with enough room for a delivery couch only) opening onto a small corridor, attending women who stay little longer six hours. If women arrive too early in the labour process, they are sent home and asked to return when nearer delivery, a time estimated by the midwives based on various physiological indicators.

Women are allocated a consultant who sets local guidelines, and has a group of medical students assigned to him. General Practitioners or the medical students and hospital housemen attend the births. Medical students are called to attend the deliveries of their respective consultants, and on occasion may be asked to deliver babies under supervision of more senior doctors or the most senior midwife. Although both medical and midwifery students must experience a certain number of deliveries to qualify for their practicing certificates, in the study hospital the medical students take precedence over midwifery students. The medical students wait in the medical teaching block, and the qualified midwives are supposed to contact them to attend immanent and essentially normal deliveries of the consultant to whom they have been allocated.

The first floor of the maternity block contains delivery suites and theatres, whilst the second and third floors are the labour wards providing for women having their first or complex births. Women who are pregnant (whose unborn child is at least twenty-four weeks old but is medically compromised) and who are being given a planned medical termination, are also given space on the third or fourth floor of the maternity block. The maternity top floors are managed by midwives who do not wear uniforms. Their ethnic identity is similar to that of the midwives in the community delivery suites on the ground floor. Midwives generally staff the top and second floors of the maternity block but obstetricians are constantly available, walking through the wards, doing rounds or ensuring that the management of their patient continues as directed.

Benjamin (1969) notes the cultural connection between capitalist social relations, work, and representations of the human body as a commodity. In medicine, head and neck surgery holds the highest status, gynaecology a lower position, and gerontology and psychiatry the lowest status within medicine. Hospitals in the UK may be structured so that they physically represent these (albeit invisible) distinctions: we see both architectural design consequences of the political power of representatives in each departments and consumer preference for high status buildings. Certainly in the study hospital, new buildings are usually for high-status surgery and obstetrics. Psychiatry and gerontology often inhabit co-opted buildings that may have been used previously as workhouses or prisons.

Treatment centres and support systems are in one large hospital setting, and may be economically sound, but the structures and service provision reinforce the status divisions within medicine. The high-status departments are clearly located at the top of the diagram (fig. 7.1): A&E, medical education, pathology and surgery. The low-status departments at the bottom: rehabilitation, elderly, nursing education, waste disposal and laundry facilities. While gynaecology is next to these, midwifery is also on the lower side of the diagram but separated from the lowest status departments by gynaecology. Its status is raised also by the fact that it occupies the most modern and newest building in the hospital, and is nearest the medical car par park and the side road leading to the hospital.

There may be a reluctance by staff to associate midwifery work with gynaecological work: the latter connotes disease, death, social terminations and failed pregnancies. Midwifery and gynaecological nursing rarely mix. Midwifery identity may also need to be maintained against the power of the obstetricians, their structural separation with higher status, and better provision of the medical as opposed to the nursing centres. Obstetricians were frequently seen by women and midwives as interfering with the normal process of childbirth. This 'women's work' in which the midwife has been 'allowed' to become expert may be acknowledged when she is permitted to support and teach the medical students about normal birth, but is undermined when medical student experience has to take precedence over midwifery student experience.

Midwives' outline of the categories for women in early pregnancy

If the practitioners are categorised, so are the mothers. The A&E Department also provides an entry point for women who are pregnant and in difficulties. The direction the women take is decided partly by the age of the foetus and the previous history of the woman. Nationally, statistics on hospital outcomes are based on successful births, on which hospital funding may also rely. Birth and death certificates, as I have said, are given if babies are twenty-four weeks or older, and/or they have breathed. In part, the structural divisions in hospital, and the placing of the women on gynaecology wards, help to manage the statistics.

Provision of services also partly meets this need: emergency scanning (within twenty-four hours) is available if the foetus is over thirteen weeks old. Prior to that, the woman is advised to go home, as miscarriage might be inevitable. At or after thirteen weeks, if the scan shows any possibility of survival, the woman will be admitted to the Early Pregnancy Unit (not available at all hospitals in the UK), for rest and assessment, otherwise she would be sent home. Women with later pregnancies (between sixteen and twenty-four weeks) are sent home to miscarry, or, if there are complications, they are admitted to gynaecology wards.

The gynaecology wards are attended by general nurses (professionals with general nurse training and qualifications) and gynaecology nurses (nurses with general training and additional specialist training in women's diseases), rather than by midwives (who have specialist knowledge of normal childbirth, the care of the mother before and after birth, and knowledge of early recognition of potential complications). The midwives I spoke to said they would go to the gynaecological ward if specifically asked. Investigations are carried out on the foetuses by pathologists only if the woman has miscarried more than four times, and through the decision of the obstetrician (fig. 7.2).

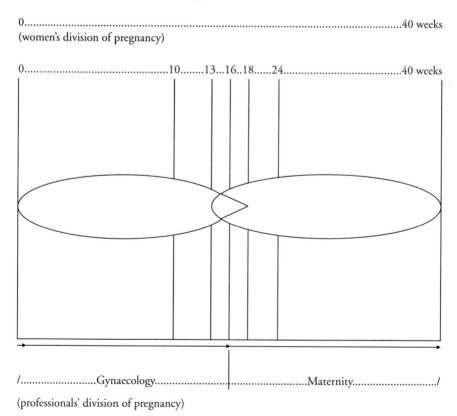

Fig 7.2 Professional delineation of pregnancy

Routine scanning of the foetus is offered only after sixteen weeks of pregnancy. Prior to that, women are offered an emergency scan (only between ten and thirteen weeks) if there is any possibility of the pregnancy being saved. Otherwise, pregnant women who come to the A&E department in labour under ten weeks' foetal age are encouraged to return home. As one midwife said:

> We send home women who are 10 weeks pregnant or less. Most people go home to have a natural miscarriage, grieving is not possible except behind curtains – we do try to fast track people through the system – and encourage them to be home.

No scanning is offered. However, from ten to thirteen weeks the woman may be admitted to a gynaecological ward as a potential surgical patient with a foetus. Scans may be offered at the higher age of the foetus of thirteen weeks. The midwife commented:

> There is a grey area from 13 weeks to 18 weeks that isn't really covered by anybody. Women who have problems before 18 weeks are sent to gynaecology. After that they have to argue a way to maternity. We have a special early pregnancy unit but the scanning department have said that is for up to 13 weeks only. We try to sneak women in and to get them scanned but we get our knuckles rapped and the patient returned if they judge her over that time, from palpation.

Another midwife, whilst sympathetic to the plight of women miscarrying, said: 'Before 18 weeks, there is no question of them going to maternity, we cannot have someone blocking a bed for ones who really need it'.

In relation to facilities on the maternity ward for late miscarriages and late medical terminations (termination of pregnancy because the child had a severe medical defect), one midwife said:

> There is no difference for us between a spontaneous miscarriage and terminations on the maternity ward for medical reasons ... there is something wrong. Not denying life as in social terminations on the gynaecology ward, but a medical decision and therefore they can openly grieve and should be together.

There is no consensus amongst the midwives about the division and provision of facilities for women in early pregnancy. Several said that the divisions added more stress and made grieving more difficult. Whilst the assumption is that going home was the 'correct' place in which to mourn, the area served by the hospital is one of high deprivation, and the midwives know that many of the women were returning to unhealthy and lonely homes. One manager remarked,

> We have a small cupboard that house records of these babies under 18 weeks, who do not survive. The records we keep contain photographs of the babies who have been dressed in clothes the woman might have provided. We arranged the baby as if sleeping. There are some nail clippings, a lock of hair, foot or handprints, printed onto card.

A small certificate written by the midwife, stating the date and time, sex if discernable, and name if given.

The preservation of these records might be the only evidence for the woman that she had borne a child. As I have said, no birth or death certificate is issued for fotuses before twenty-four weeks. The midwives say that women who loses a child often does not visit again for some time. Then, they would often come in to find the midwife who had delivered their child that had 'died', and look at the midwifery records. The parents interviewed said that they were unable to face the 'death' at the time but that they were grateful that something had been kept, which had kept the child alive for them.

The paediatrician from the midwife's viewpoint

The midwives whom I interviewed emphasised consumer choice (rather than professional control) in regard to giving birth. Midwives said they acted as the woman's advocate concerning her right to choose, say, birth position, the administration of pain-controlling medication, or the regularity of vaginal examinations. In doing so they sometimes counteract local guidelines formulated by obstetricians, and reinforce the midwife's professional judgment and actions. As one midwife said:

Very often guidelines on the labour ward will differ from consultant to consultant ... For example, the woman's consultant may want a more actively managed labour (for example vaginal examination will be done at hourly intervals each woman will be monitored like this throughout labour) . If the midwife works these guidelines it restricts the possibility of her ability to say to the woman 'do you feel like walking round'. 'Do you feel like taking up a different position?' Again it's a balance because the midwife is supposed to be the lead professional when it comes to dealing with low risk mothers during labour, so really the midwife should be free to make the decisions. In reality where she must do it and why this or that hasn't been done is often questioned by the obstetrician. But there is this influence in being seen to work alongside these guidelines, and really in the labour ward, in the modern labour ward there is a continued presence of the obstetric staff consultants who will come in and say why hasn't this been done or that been done. It has to be a very assertive midwife who says 'this is what the woman wants and this is how we want to conduct this labour'. Even though the midwife's professional judgments might predominate in a normal birth, there is also a range of the abnormal births that she feels she could deal with before having recourse to the obstetrician: If everything is going well you don't need the obstetrician telling you what to do. For example when a woman was in labour and contracting at a rate I thought she should contract the only problem was the meconium stained liquor[2] which we know that if nothing else happens, unless the baby's heart rate gets worse and signs of the baby getting distressed, there is no need for constant intervention from obstetrician. I knew the woman was asking good progress and would deliver in good course.

Another midwife discussed the usual procedures and baseline measure, and her role in deciding to involve the doctor or not.

> We welcome the mother, take temperatures first, if membranes are ruptured we monitor everything initially as a baseline, and the activity of the baby on admission of the woman and we can print the information off usually for 30 minutes. If during the observation something goes wrong, or veers towards the abnormal you can put that woman back on the monitor and compare it with the admission readings, you read it and see whether to involve the doctor or not.

Concerns about the physiological aspect of the birth, and medical intervention, were often expressed in discussions. As another midwife remarked:

> Purely in the high risk cases we are quite prepared to let the doctor say what they want in the high risk area that is their realm, we have to adhere to what they want and we have to know what to give ... But when it comes to a normal vaginal delivery they know what to do throughout their training they know what they should do and what they should not. There is fear of rupturing the membrane, the midwife would like the woman to rupture by herself , but the doctor would see the membranes as having no functional use beyond three centimetres. If you break the waters and then if the contractions stops they put up a drip, and then ... once the intervention starts the whole thing cascades right up to the woman being on the theatre table for that particular period of time.

Whilst the medical presence is there constantly, midwives can still assert some control and emphasise autonomy of practice:

> Absolutely, particularly with the normal vaginal delivery, and this autonomy varies from unit to unit. If this unit is a very high 'midwife's unit' the doctors do not interfere, the midwives will not let them interfere. In fact there are cases where you are in the room and the doctor knocks on the door and you say everything is fine and he walks on. Where as you go to another unit and you find it is a very highly technically managed unit where the doctor will always want to know everything that is going on, and will almost turn that woman into an abnormal person, an ill woman. Whereas we see women as doing physiological things that are not abnormal, so there is always this debate going on between the doctors and midwives about them eroding the midwives' autonomy.

Midwives on other midwives

In the UK, at the turn of the century, the midwife was still firmly associated with the domestic scene, as more than 95 percent of births were at home. By 1945, the profession had become institutionalised, and almost 60 percent of confinements were hospital births, (OPCS 1974–85; OPCS 1985; RCOG 1982; Registrar

General 1972). The pharmacological treatment of haemolytic streptococci, the primary cause of sepsis, radically reduced the maternal mortality rate. The recognition and treatment of toxaemia to prevent major fits (eclampsia), and then rapid recognition and response to pre- and post-partum haemorrhage reduced further maternal deaths. There have been extensive debates about the impact of medical intervention in maternity care (Health Statistics Quarterly 2003; Campbell and Macfarlane 1987; Sinclair *et al.* 1981). Indeed, the use of continuous foetal monitoring (CFM) which aims to reduce perinatal mortality and cerebral palsy, has been scrutinised recently by NICE (2001) in its review of the literature and a meta-analysis of the randomised controlled trials researching the subject. NICE's finding suggest that CFM did not support any impact on the aims, and worse, showed increased medical intervention associated with its use. Internationally, a country's standing may be influenced significantly by levels of maternal and infant mortality. In the UK, various government departments of public health conduct close and regular reviews of maternal and infant mortality and morbidity. Indeed, all UK hospitals have to provide statistics showing outcomes in different departments, and have specific targets they need to reach in order to be remunerated (Health Care Commission 2004). As we have already seen, this may have profound implications for the expectant, labouring or nursing mother because of space and staffing implications.

In an earlier paper on midwife identity in the same study hospital, I demonstrated a gender elision in reproduction that has led to more egalitarian procreativity (Littlewood 2003). However, although the actual physical effort of giving birth might be made more pain-free, and more egalitarian with the involvement of male partners, birth still presents some disjunctures and difficulties that question the midwives' identity. Their position is one of being 'by and for women', that birth is physiological and will happen 'regardless', and that the essence of good midwifery is both the physical integrity of the perineum, the woman, and the safe delivery of the child.

An ethnography of the hospital, however, suggests that hierarchical rather than egalitarian modes operate in the delivery room, processes that may be as much for reasons of professional protectionism, as for the need to reinforce gender differences to protect the labouring woman. Of real interest is how descriptions of the midwife's position are maintained as an autonomous practitioner in relation to the obstetrician and the husband against a backdrop of 'risk culture'.

Two midwives discussed the difficulty of acting with too much autonomy. Sometimes midwives will not support each other, unlike doctors, who are perceived as being extremely supportive of each other. As one midwife said:

> having said that you have to be very good as deciding when you want the doctor to intervene or when you don't want the doctor to intervene, and use your own clinical judgment based on the UKCC Code of Practice and make sure when you decide what to do that you were right; and that is why midwives shy away from this as they will be held accountable for things going wrong, and it is not uncommon for some midwives

to toe the line because of litigation, and work as doctor's handmaids just to not being named and blamed for unforeseen circumstances.

Another midwife helped to clarify further the division between the obstetricians and the midwives:

> Yes, in any unit there are guidelines … but in my last unit the guidelines were dominated by midwifery. Midwives wrote it and it goes to whatever committee and it is implemented. Whereas, you may go to another place and the consultant presides over the committee, and it is just that the guidelines from committee outcome reflect how strong the midwifery manager is and what is the game of midwifery and the game of obstetrics and how well they can argue their place.

Observing midwives in action

Midwives are recognised on the basis of a variety of qualifications: through diploma or degree courses, by direct entry studying midwifery only, or by studying midwifery after nursing. In the UK, midwives have many choices as to where they work. Their locations include private hospitals, National Health Service hospitals, in the community in group practices or General Practitioner practices, at birth centres, as independent groups, or as part of integrated twenty-four-hour care. The units in which they work may be led by consultants, general practitioners, or by midwives. Within the UK they were the first professional group that had to undergo continuing examined assessments throughout their professional life. If they wish to practise, UK law obliges them to register with the National Register of Midwives. Also, by UK law, a qualified practitioner (physician or midwife) must attend deliveries. Planned home deliveries must be sanctioned by a qualified practitioner, who must agree to be present at the birth.

Following the government report *Changing Childbirth* (1993), couple-centred delivery was advocated to encourage paternal involvement. Partners are now actively encouraged by the obstetricians in the hospital to stay throughout the birth. The study hospital had guidelines that paralleled these changes nationally. Having a partner present provides continuity for the woman in the increasing fragmentation of NHS service. It also acknowledges that shared activity is possible with an increasingly aware and educated public. The general effects of these changes were that midwives encouraged women and their partners to have a birth plan that they could all work with for the delivery. The driving forces in the government documents have been economic, support, and the delegation of some activities to the partners in a normal delivery. Because of reduced staff, the midwife may be involved in delivering more than one woman at a time; thus, the working co-operation of a partner becomes essential.

In the main study we traced the pathways of women who came to hospital in labour, and looked at how the different professionals were drawn into the work. Midwives, of course, do not work alone in hospitals. The following example illuminates the various medical identities involved in a typical case. Whilst comments about roles and differences are frequent in everyday practice and in quiet times, at points of crisis, individual practitioners slide into action with well defined paths, enhancing care at critical times for the patient, or in this case the woman, her husband and the twins.

On one particular occasion, the duty midwife in the maternity block had been rung up by a casualty sister and asked to go to casualty. When she walked over, a twenty-year-old woman had arrived at A&E with her husband; she had recently moved into the catchment area and had no previous contact with the hospital. The woman had been placed in a cubicle while the nurse sent for a midwife and casualty officer. The casualty officer examined the woman, and requested the presence of an obstetric registrar. The midwife rang the midwifery manager in the maternity block, and contacted the medical students as well as the student midwives in the nursing and medical education centres. The woman was thirty weeks pregnant and was in premature labour, expecting twins. An intravenous infusion was put up by the obstetric registrar. After two hours in casualty, the woman was transferred to the maternity block. An ambulance was requested, but none was available, so the woman was placed on a trolley bed. Porters were requested. A porter, midwife, nurse, medical student and the husband wheeled the woman along the corridors of the hospital, down in a lift, onto the pavement, and past the bus stop.

A student midwife joined the group, with two other medical students. One of the medical students went ahead and stopped the traffic in the hospital whilst the trolley was pushed onto the road. The nurse held an umbrella over the woman and a medical student put his coat over her. The group reached the maternity building, walked the twenty yards along the ground floor to the lifts, and took the lift to the third floor maternity unit to be joined by the midwifery manager.

The midwife and student midwives transferred the woman from the trolley to a bed near the ward desk, and the curtains were pulled round. The midwife, with the medical student, attached two straps around the woman's tummy, from a machine that allowed visual and sound recording of the baby's heart. The midwife showed the medical student how to feel for the baby, and to listen using a foetal stethoscope. A medical student under instructions from the obstetric registrar put up another intravenous infusion with medication. The midwife answered the husband's questions and showed student midwives how to feel and listen for the woman's pregnancy.

The obstetrician came in and listened. He told the woman she was in premature labour and that one of the twins was lying horizontally. The medication was to try to stop the contractions, but as yet it had not, and the twins might be in danger. There was a real possibility that she would have to undergo an operation to get them out. The obstetrician then contacted the anaesthetist, and paediatricians in case there was a need for an emergency delivery. The ward sister contacted theatre sisters to make them aware of the case and give an approximate time of arrival and the potential problems. The woman was crying, and the midwife asked the student midwife to take the husband outside as he was feeling sick. One medical student was looking after the foetal monitoring machine, the other medical students and midwifery student stood silent in the background. The obstetrician explained that a caesarean section might be necessary and explained the procedure and gave the consent (a form which has to be signed by the woman, patient or guardian of anyone undergoing an operation in the UK) form to the midwife to complete with the woman.

The anaesthetist came in and asked questions about food, allergies, previous medical history, and other children. The woman said she felt wet. The midwife examined her and found her waters had broken and were stained with faeces, sometimes a sign of increased distress of the unborn baby. The foetal heart rate had increased again for one of the twins. The obstetrician decided it would not be wise to wait any longer, and went off to theatre to prepare for the operation. The midwife disconnected the woman from the foetal monitor; no porters were available, so she was wheeled in her bed to the operating theatre by the medical students, anaesthetist, and midwife. The husband walked with them to the lift and walked one floor down to the theatre with a medical student, where the theatre staff and two paediatricians were waiting. The obstetrician was in theatre scrubbing up. The midwife took the husband to the relatives' room, and the students went into the observation room over the theatre. The midwife explained everything to the husband again. He requested a priest, whom the midwife contacted. Within half an hour, the theatre staff came to say that he had a healthy baby boy, but the second twin, also a boy, had died. The midwife took the husband to see his live son, who was in an incubator. He then was taken to his wife, who was in the recovery room.

The obstetrician discussed with the parents the need to have a post-mortem on the baby who had died, and that the baby needed to go to pathology as soon as possible. The midwife talked with them about their son who had died; both wished to see him. The midwives had washed the baby, whom the parents held, and the midwife took a photograph. She then covered the baby's foot with coloured ink and took a print, and took a print of the baby's hand. Having received consent to carry out the post-mortem, the midwife rang the porters to ask them to collect the baby for pathology. The baby was placed in a coffin that was placed within a basket by the midwife. This was then carried by the porter and accompanied by a student midwife to pathology.

The midwife explained to the husband that the baby would go from there to the hospital mortuary, and that certificates for the baby would be provided by the doctors. These the husband would take to the Registrar of Births and Deaths in the Patient Services Department at the hospital, which would issue a release form for the baby from the mortician where the baby would go after pathology, but the baby might remain with the pathologists for two or three days. The husband asked to go with the baby to pathology. The midwife allocated a student midwife and medical student to be with the husband – who had now been in the hospital for over ten hours – to sort out transport for him to go home, or to contact relatives, and to obtain a hot drink for him as there were no vending machines for relatives in the maternity block. The midwife then sat with the woman, listening to her, helping to show her how to breastfeed her new baby.

Core players	Others
Expectant woman	General physicians (casualty officers)
Midwifery tutors	Gynaecologists
Hospital midwives	Scanners
Student midwives	Anaesthetists
Community midwives	Pathologists
General practitioners	Counselors
Medical students	Managers
Obstetricians	Nurses (A&E and theatres)
Partners/family	Theatre staff (technicians)
Babies	Porters
	Paediatricians
	Mortician and Registrar

7.3 Potential agents in each obstetric management

In the above case, at least nineteen different professionals were involved in the management of just one mother (The full complement of agents who might conceivably be involved are schematized in fig. 7.3.) UK government documents argue for teamwork within and between professionals, and a partnership in care between professionals and consumers. In this crisis, for example, we see how the midwife's identity slipped seamlessly into that of clinical practitioner, educator, facilitator and teacher.

Discussion of midwifery identity

Benjamin (1969) explores the idea of social relations work on the human body, drawing from the lack of distinction between work and labour in Marx's thought. We can conceive of labour as the physical exchange, whereas work is the social process through which humanity creates durable objects and relations. We are embedded in the symbolic orderly language of communication, and intrinsic culturally formative activity of work and therefore identity. Work, therefore shifts social consciousness, from one largely derivative of the logic of production, to culture, the communicative practice of differently positioned human subjects.

Ulin (2002) shows how work and self-identity are instrumental acts in relation to nature, transforming identity into acts of differentiated cultural production. Midwives, for example, have not only to *own*, but also to *re-naturalise* labour. The delivery of a new infant is now a '*non- natural* product', a product of high technology and obstetrics. Identity comes from individual appropriation. Midwives reinterpret their craft by attempting to offer 'normal' home conditions within a hospital setting (birth cushions, partners, allowing the woman to walk around, or use different birth positions), trying to reproduce a natural outcome. However high-tech 'obstetrics', science and the creeping changes in the structural organisation of the hospital, its policy and economic control over labour, insinuate into the pregnant woman's experience of the new life.

From the previous pages, we can see the emerging identity of the midwife in reference to four areas of discussion: physical structure, categorisation, space, and moral and social silence.

Physical structure

Reproduction of the social order occurs in the microcosm of the hospital. As I have noted, the physical structure of the hospital reflects status divisions. Within the hospital there is an attempt to maintain a static, timeless order by routine, hierarchy, and strict maintenance of the position of objects (beds, bed wheels, etc). Midwives in the study appear similar in that they have uniforms, understand the status of the different areas in which they work, and realise the fragility of their attempts to be independent practitioners, as they may become bereft of peer support should an infant death occur (derived from ideas in Harrison 1992, 1999, 2002). Their shared cultural concern, i.e., the care of the patient, unless at points of real crisis, is not necessarily a source of cohesion (Gluckman 1977; Helgason and Palsson 1997) or politeness (Hendry 1989).

Although she is likened to a 'ritual specialist' in some societies (Rasmussen 1992), the midwife in the UK is someone who now must very quickly guide and shape the labouring women and their partners, in their very short experience of the midwife's space: the hospital labour room (Gineratnu 2001). After many years of ongoing debate, midwives remain the symbolic property of the doctor (Hirschon 1984) who prescribes their role, to deliver only 'normal births', whether in the hospital or at home (Marsh 1985; Tew 1985; 1986; WHO 1985; Kitzinger and Davis 1978; Kerr *et al.* 1954). Statistics and risk prediction scores and assessments have been used to tighten control of where, when, and how childbirth should be managed (Charmers *et al.* 1989; Hall *et al.* 1985, Sinclair *et al.* 1981; Butler and Alberman 1969). The ethics of professional interference in childbirth and its medical consequences have been explored (Zander 1981); likewise, various governments and medical departments have used the clear relationship between poverty and poor birth outcome (Black *et al.* 1980) to support increased hospitalization and technological intervention by medical professionals. We see this clearly, for example, in the rise of caesarian births in the UK.

In relation to the division between obstetrics and gynaecology, the latter has a longer tradition within medicine, being identified as a legitimate sub-speciality of surgery well established in the UK as early as 1900. Obstetrics, by contrast, did not have a distinct official identity – nor college, with formal separate approval – until nearly thirty years later, when a joint medical degree Diploma was awarded in Obstetrics and Gynaecology. Nearly a further twenty years passed before a separate Diploma in Obstetrics was awarded, confirming status, standards and proficiency. Similar standards were developed for the midwife in the UK, culminating in various Acts of Parliament defining the qualifications and standards required of midwives attending women in labour. An example is the Midwives' Act 1902 to 1926, and then 1936, that also influenced British Dominions (RCOM 1987; Shaw 1954).

As noted above, practising midwives in the UK, as in many cultures, grew from the notion of 'wise women' or 'with woman', a helper in events seen as 'women's business' dealing with women at all points of their lives, and especially during and after childbirth (Towler and Bramall 1986). From these more general beginnings, the role of the midwife has become gradually more restricted and specialised: medical advances, and especially the professionalisation of physicians, have removed activities from the control of midwives. Midwives remain part of the doctor's team, with very few able to set up practice independent of medical control. These latter are very expensive, private midwife services that are still obliged to inform the woman's physician of their activities. Whilst many UK midwives might wish to carry out one-to-one care throughout pregnancy and birth, serious staff shortages, and poor midwifery support, make this a reality only to the smallest minority of the country.

Categorisation

Of concern to the midwives in this study is the professional division of the pregnancy, and the division of care between maternity and gynaecology departments. Termination of pregnancy for social reasons takes place in gynaecology departments. As we have seen, there may be no official marker for the woman that her baby has died; the life of the terminated baby receives little acknowledgment. Here the woman is often in the hospital as a 'day case', sometimes staying only a few hours before going home. On the other hand. where there is a medical problem with the baby, and a termination has been recommended or requested, the life of the unborn baby is acknowledged. This takes place on the maternity ward, where mourning for this category of death can be public and open. Although categorisation is useful to manage information to maximum efficiency, it has the unforeseen effects of finely controlling how life itself is defined. Women become aware that strenuous efforts to prolong a pregnancy will not be made if they are admitted to a gynaecology ward (Littlewood 1999). Pregnant women are admitted to the top-floor maternity building only if over twenty-four weeks in pregnancy. From a lay perspective, as the duration of pregnancy is forty weeks, equal attention and equivalence of 'life' throughout might be expected. In fact, the forty weeks is 'chunked up' statistically by the organisation, where the woman is directed to A&E, special units, gynaecology or home, depending on the age of the pregnancy, but guided away from maternity until beyond the twenty-four week barrier. Finally, the midwife has to retain her identity as 'expert' in the birth situation where consumer choice has led to a woman undergoing difficult labour, along with the participation of her partner (Levine 1999). The midwife is not expected to give any personal views of the partnership, the woman's status, the origin of the baby, and how the newborn and parents fit into the social order. To be considered 'perfect', the birth event ideally should remain narrowly focused on physiological considerations.

In the study, midwives stated that the woman's race appeared to make no difference; 'problem women' were not identified by their colour, age, or partner. Likewise, the acceptance of the partner in the delivery room with the labouring woman was least difficult if the partner acted not as advocate for the woman, but as an adjunct to the midwife, reinforcing what she saw as her identity, i.e., working with the midwife to produce a healthy live baby. Within the hospital, self-identity was reinforced by the structure of the hospital, and the way in which different departments facilitated or limited discussion of the midwife's role. Further, the consequence of the symbolic primacy of midwifery over gynaecology is the separation of women's illness and other issues. These separations affect the 'cut-off' points of new life and how the hospital services react to it because of the structure. The structural provision of scanning the pregnant woman controls the midwives' decision-making, and thereby the pathways left open to the midwife for the care of the woman. The service categorisation ensures midwifery is associated with life; anything else is separated off at arbitrary points.

Space

In the study hospital, midwives are physically separated from other nurses in a similar professional area. They are also separated from labouring women because of the increasingly short time in contact with the midwife. However they are also separated from others hierarchically as well as spatially. The idea of space as a 'field of relations' (Olwig and Hastrup 1997), rather than as 'theories of practice' (Bhaskar 1979; Bourdieu 1977), has been used to understand social relations. Space as a form of classifying territory from a Durkheimian position has been used effectively in understanding social relations (Gell 1992; Ardener 1981; Levi-Strauss 1966). 'Field of relations', the myriad social relationships with peers, team practitioners and the labouring women and their partners, is a way in which the midwife may gain 'capacity' (the accruing of power, information and support for personal or work changes). However, because of the narrowing of her occupational focus and the increasing technology within childbirth, she is separated from this potential power that might give her a stronger identity.

Social and moral silence

Although claiming a neutral position in regard to the labouring woman about moral and ethical issues, midwives nevertheless raised concerns personally about the gender of partners, in vitro fertilisation, surrogacy, and silent incest, wondering 'where will it all end?' (issues raised in Konrad 1998; Mosko 1992; Rival 1998; Levi-Strauss 1969; Oakes et al. 1994; Oakes 1987). Space as 'capacity', as the moral and ethical ground rules shift, becomes more elastic. Known kinship patterns, expected boundaries of incest relations (Edwards 2002), gender and religious affiliation because of technological advances, have further reduced the midwife's 'capacity', where she now keeps a moral and social silence on the possible implications for the new baby in the social structure.

Critical understanding of work and identity requires a theoretical framework that is attentive to norms. Viewing work as a cultural production shifts the emphasis in Marxism from 'social consciousness' – largely derivative of the logic of production – to culture as a communicative process involving differently positioned subjects. Policy, guidelines, laws, and statistical cut-off points reinforce this structural streamlining. Consumers now expect that up-to-date medical dominance and technology 'cannot fail', and have accepted them, trusting that the change in laws governing midwifery practice and encouraging first births in hospital, will maintain good statistical outcomes. To produce a 'natural' new life, free from stigma involving gender peculiarities (only white cards are now held up to show a birth, pink or blue having been seen as too formative), the origin of sperm (partners of any sex, not fathers only, are now encouraged to be present), or the origin of the egg (non-biological birth-mother, mothers producing babies for non-family members, grandmothers and sisters having their relative's child), requires reduced participation of the midwife in the social birth of the child.

Although managing her identity within the hospital hierarchy, at the point of birth, the midwife is likely to assume a neutral identity for the mother to manage the micropolitics of a new social being. The baby is now declared 'a baby', no longer declared a boy or a girl', but is handed over to the woman who may or may not be the biological mother, or have the presence and support of the biological father. Indeed, the father may be a surrogate, a same-sex partner, or possibly a website identity. Any or all of these alternative social arrangements may produce new challenges for the midwife in the development of her identity through social relationships.

Conclusion

The role of the midwife, in relation to the pregnant woman and child, is a highly contested area. The current mode of care is the result of historical changes, and the narrowing of the midwife's role and, indeed, identity. Midwifery identity is fragile: its construction within the hospital is bound up with the ever-changing way we define life itself. Scanning shows life at younger and younger foetal stages, but this has led to arguments that the service cannot provide a full range of maternity requirements in hospital, and cut-off points have to be made. Thus, midwifery identity is subject to contestation and the play of shifting historical, political, economic and cultural grounds.

As I have noted, the wealth of a country is often assumed to correlate with its maternal and infant mortality figures; thus, policy regarding the support and care of labouring women in hospital has become more and more closely regulated where monies for health provision to maternity hospital are directly related to target goals. Pregnancy is statistically 'chunked up' to try to remove 'failed births' from the official records of 'live births'. Pregnant women are encouraged to have miscarriages at home, are diverted to gynaecology wards if there is no hope of the unborn baby surviving, sent to specialist high-risk units for difficult or unpredictable deliveries and outcomes, as well as screened earlier and with separate provision made for abnormalities in both the mother and the child. Because of the channelling of pregnancy and birth, midwives increasingly focus only on the live, 'perfect' baby. Their independent status is a double-edged sword, where they mutually support each other in this focus, but are left isolated and fearful if anything goes wrong. The likelihood of things going wrong is reduced because maternity provision has stricter controls over antenatal care and qualified practitioner intervention. But if things do go amiss, there are detailed and intense inquiries where individual practitioners are named and held accountable.

In the UK, the identity of midwives is forged through a narrowing of policy, and the institutional attempt to 'remove' or manage death. This process has resulted in a reduced moral or social role for midwives, but an enormous increase in the professional legitimacy of their identity within the hospital. The midwife is now much less symbolically associated with the protection of the child within the community. Her identity is increasingly bound up in the technologically and bureaucratically rationalised birth of a viable baby; however, its right to life through technology has the unintended consequence of making the midwife's own identity increasingly invisible.

Acknowledgements

I gratefully acknowledge the helpful comments on the manuscript provided by Dr S. Ardener, OBE, and Professor K. Maynard.

Notes

1. The figures for maternity unit deliveries, induction rate, caesarian rate, instrument delivery and normal birth rate, and whether the units are consultant, doctor or midwife-led ones, are recorded in BirthChoiceUK maternity statistics (BCUK 2003). Unemployment is 6 percent (London 7 percent); it has the highest birth rate per 1,000 population (with 16.3, compared with 14.8 for London and 12.3 for England as a whole). Births for age

group 15–44 are 70.91 live births/1,000 women (compared with the London figure of 63.56). Stillbirth rates are 5.8 per 1,000 total births (compared with London 6.2, and England 5.3). Thirty-five percent of the populations are black and minority ethnic groups (6th highest percentage in London). The abortion/miscarriage rates per 1000 women for the 16–19 year age group, 32.2 compared with England 24.6); for the 20–4 year age group, 48.8 (England 29.2); for the 25–34 year olds, 9.6 (England 17.2), for the 35–39 years olds, 16.1 (England 8.9). Further indices of deprivation are the percentage of births under 1500 g forming 1.6 (compared with 1.5 for London as a whole), and under 2500 gs 8.3 percent (compared with the figure for London of 8.1 percent). In the study year, just half the births were 'normal births', 28.6 percent were caesarian (compared with a national average of 21 percent, 17.2 percent induced, 6.2 percent instrument delivery (NHS Maternity Statistics 2000–2001, BirthChoiceUK 2004).

2. If distressed, the baby may pass faecal matter in the womb. This is an early sign, and may be a serious one, that the baby is getting into difficulties, and urgent action in completing the birth needs to be considered. It is usually accompanied by a very high or very low foetal heart rate.

References

Ardener, S. (ed.). 1981. *Women and Space: Ground Rules and Social Maps.* London: Croom Helm.

Benjamin, W. 1969. *Illumination.* New York: Schocken Books.

Bhaskar, R. 1979. *The Possibility of Naturalism: A Philosophical Critique of the Contemporary Human Sciences.* Brighton: Harvester.

BirthChoiceUK. 2004. *Maternity Statistics for 2002.* www.birthchoiceuk.com/hospitals.

Black, D., J. Morris, C. Smith and P. Townsend. 1980. *Inequalities in Health.* The Black Report. Middlesex: Penguin Books.

Bloch, M. 1992. *Prey into Hunter: The Politics of Religious Experience.* Cambridge: Cambridge University Press.

Bourdieu, P. 1977. *Outline of a Theory of Practice.* Cambridge: Cambridge University Press.

Brunton, R. 1989. 'The Cultural Instability of Egalitarian Societies'. *Man* (n.s.) 24: 673–81.

Butler, N., and E. Alberman (eds). 1969. *Perinatal Problems.* Edinburgh: Livingstone.

Campbell, R., and A. Macfarlane. 1987. *Where to be Born? The Debate and the Evidence.* Oxford: National Perinatal Epidemiology Unit.

Charmers, I., M. Enkin, M and M. Keirse (eds). 1989. *Effective Care in Pregnancy and Childbirth.* Oxford: Oxford University Press.

Department of Health 1970. *The Peel Report.* London: HMSO.

Durham, D. 1995. 'Soliciting Gifts and Negotiating Agency: The Spirit of Asking in Botswana'. *Journal of the Royal Anthropological Institute* 1: 111–28.

Edwards, J. 2002. 'Incorporating Incest: Gamete, Body and Relation in Assisted Conception'. *The Journal of the Royal Anthropological Institute* (n.s.) 10: 755–74.

Gell, A. 1992. *The Anthropology of Time: Cultural Constructions of Temporal Maps and Images.* Oxford: Berg.

Gillison, G. 1980. 'Images of Nature in Gimi Thought'. In *Nature, Culture, Gender.* C. MacCormack and M. Strathern (eds). Cambridge: Cambridge University Press.

Gineratnu, A. 2001. 'Shaping the Tourist's Gaze: Representing Ethnic Difference in a Nepali Village'. *Journal of the Royal Anthropological Institute* (n.s.) 7: 527–43.

Gluckman, M. 1977. *Politics, Law and Ritual in Tribal Society.* Oxford: Blackwell.

Hall, M., S. MacKintyre and M. Porter. 1985. *Antenatal Care Assessed.* Aberdeen: Aberdeen University Press.

Hansard, House of Commons. 2004. NHS Statistics (London), *Qualified Midwives in the London Government Office Region by Organization and Contract.* www.parliament. co.uk/cm200304.

Harrison, S.J. 1992. 'Ritual as Intellectual Property'. *Man* (n.s.) 27: 225–44.

_____ 1999. 'Identity as a Scarce Resource'. *Social Anthropology* 7: 239–51.

_____ 2002. 'The Politics of Resemblance: Ethnicity Trademarks, Head Hunting'. *Man* (n.s.) 8: 211–32.

Health Care Commission. 2004. *The Health and Social Care (Community Health and Standards) Act 2003.* www.healthcarecommission.org.uk.

Health Statistics Quarterly. 2003. *Infant and Perinatal Mortality by Social and Biological Factors.* www.statistics.gov.uk/releases.

Helgason, A. and G. Palsson. 1997. 'Contested Commodities: the Moral Landscape of Modernist Regimes'. *Journal of the Royal Anthropological Institute* (n.s.) 3: 451–71.

Hendry, J. 1989. 'To Wrap or Not to Wrap: Politeness and Penetration in Ethnographic Enquiry'. *Man* (n.s.) 24(4): 620–35.

Hirschon, R. (ed.). 1984. *Women and Property-Women as Property.* London: Croom Helm.

James, W. 1977. '*Placing the Unborn: On the Social Construction of New Life*'. Kaberry Memorial Lecture (ms), University of Oxford.

Jarman. B. 1983. 'Identification of Underprivileged Areas'. *British Medical Journal* (Clin Res Ed) May 28, 286 (6379) 1705–9.

_____ 1984. 'Underprivileged Areas Validation and Distribution Scores'. *British Medical Journal,* (Clin Res Ed) Dec 8, 289 (6458) 1587–92.

Kerr, M.J.M., R.W. Johnstone and M.H. Phillips. 1954. *Historical Review of Obstetrics and Gynaecology 1800–1950.* Edinburgh: Livingstone.

Kitzinger, S. and J. Davis (eds). 1978. *The Place of Birth.* Oxford: Oxford University Press.

Konrad, M. 1998. 'Ova Donation and Symbols of Substance: Some Variations on the Theme of Sex, Gender and the Partible Person'. *Journal of the Royal Anthropological Institute* 4(4): 643–68.

Levine, H.B. 1999. 'Reconstructing Ethnicity'. *Journal of the Royal Anthropological Institute* (n.s.) 5: 165–80.

Lévi-Strauss, C. 1966. *Structural Anthropology.* New York: Basic Books.

_____ 1969. *The Elementary Structures of Kinship.* Boston: Beacon Press.

Littlewood, J. 1999. 'From an Invisibility of Miscarriage to an Understanding of Life'. *Anthropology and Medicine* 6: 217–30.

_____ 2000. *Mortuary Rituals for a Nobody.* Seminar Series: Death and Identity. Oxford: Institute of Social and Cultural Anthropology, University of Oxford.

_____ 2003. *The Ambiguity of Labour: The Identity of Midwives.* Seminar Series: Ethnicity and Identity. Oxford: Institute of Social and Cultural Anthropology, University of Oxford.

MacCormack, C. and M. Strathern (eds). 1980. *Nature, Culture, Gender.* Cambridge: Cambridge University Press.

Marsh, G.N. (ed.) 1985. *Introduction to Modern Obstetrics in General Practice.* Oxford: Oxford University Press.

Mosko, M. 1992. 'Motherless Sons: "Divine Kings" and "Partible Persons" in Melanesia and Polynesia'. *Man* (n.s.) 27(4): 697–717.

National Institute for Clinical Excellence (NICE). 2001. *The Use of Electronic Foetal Monitoring.* London: HMSO

NHS Maternity Statistics. 2004. *Maternity Statistics for England 1998–99 to 2000–01.* www.pub.doh.gov.uk/pub.sb0211.

Oakes, P. 1987. *The Salience of Social Categories.* In *Rediscovering the Social Group, eds* B. Turner et al. Oxford: Basil Blackwell.

Oakes, P., S. Haslam and J. Turner. 1994. *Stereotyping and Social Reality.* Oxford: Basil Blackwell.

Office of Population Census and Surveys (OPCS). 1974–85 *Statistical Review.* London: OPCS.

Olwig, K.F. and K. Hastrup (eds). 1997. *Siting Culture: The Shifting Anthropological Object.* London: Routledge.

Rasmussen, S. 1992. 'Ritual Specialists, Ambiguity and Power in Tuareg Society'. *Man* (n.s.) 27: 105–28.

Registrar General. 1972. *Statistical Review for England and Wales.* London: HMSO.

Rival, L. 1998. 'Androgynous Parents and Guest Children: The Huaorani Couvade'. *Journal of the Royal Anthropological Institute* 4: 619–42.

Robertson, A.F. 1996. 'The Development of Meaning: Ontogeny and Culture'. *Journal of the Royal Anthropological Institute* (n.s.) 2: 591–610.

Royal College of Gynaecologists (RCOG). 1982. *A Place of Birth.* London: Royal College of Gynaecologists.

Royal College of Midwives (RCOM). 1987. *The Role and Education of the Future Midwife in the United Kingdom.* London: Royal College of Midwives.

Shaw, W.F. 1954. *Twenty-Five Years. The Story of the Royal College of Obstetricians and Gynaecologist 1929–1954.* London: Churchill.

Sinclair, J., G. Torrance, M. Boyle, et al. 1981. 'Evaluation of Neonatal-intensive-care Programs'. *New England Journal of Medicine* 305: 489–93.

Strathern, M. 1988. *The Gender of the Gift: Problems with Women and Problems with Society in Melanesia.* Berkeley: University of California Press.

Strathern, M. 1992. *Reproducing the Future: Anthropology, Kinship and the New Reproductive Technologies.* Manchester: Manchester University Press.

—————— 1996. 'Cutting the Network'. *The Journal of the Royal Anthropological Institute* (n.s) 2: 517–35.

Tajfel, H. 1981. *Human Groups and Social Categories.* Cambridge: Cambridge University Press.

Tew, M. 1985. 'Place of Birth and Peri-natal Mortality'. *Journal of the Royal College of General Practitioners* 35: 390–4.

—————— 1986. 'Do Obstetric Intranatal Interventions Make Birth Safer?' *British Journal of Obstetrics and Gynaecology* 93: 659–74.

Toren, C. [1996] 1999. 'Compassion for One Another: Constituting Kinship as Intensionality in Fiji'. *The Journal of the Royal Anthropological Institute.* (n.s) 5: 265–80.

Towler, J. and J. Bramell. 1986. *Midwives in History and Society.* London: Croom Helm.

Townsend, P., P. Phillmore and A. Beattie. 1988. *Health and Deprivation: Inequalities and the North.* London: Croom Helm.

Ulin, R.C. 2002. 'Work as a Cultural Production: Labour and Self Identity Among Southwest French Wine Growers'. *The Journal of the Royal Anthropological Institute* (n.s.) 8: 691–712.

Whitehouse, H. 1996. 'Rites of Terror: Emotion, Metaphor and Memory in Melanesian Initiation Cults'. *The Journal of the Royal Anthropological Institute* (n.s.) 2: 703–15.

World Health Organisation (WHO). 1985. *Having a Baby in Europe: Public Health in Europe.* 26. Geneva: WHO.

Zander, L. 1981. 'The Place of Confinement: a Question of Statistics or Ethics?'. *Journal of Medical Ethics* 7(3): 123–7.

NOTES ON CONTRIBUTORS

Gina Buijs is Professor of Anthropology and Development Studies, and is the Assistant Vice-Rector: Academic at the University of Zululand, KwaZulu-Natal, South Africa. She has lectured in social anthropology at various universities in South Africa, and has been a Visiting Research Fellow at the Centre for Cross-Cultural Research on Women (now the International Gender Studies Centre) at Queen Elizabeth House, University of Oxford. Her research interests include religion, gender, migration and ethnicity as well as rural development issues. Among her edited books is Migrant Women (Berg 1993, reprinted 1995).

Janette Davies is a Member of the International Gender Studies Centre and a Research Associate at Queen Elizabeth House, Department for International Development, University of Oxford. A former health worker in Bolivia, Cambodia and Bangladesh, her present research focuses on dying with dignity, ageing and dying amidst technology. She is currently working on a book entitled, Life Before Death: quality of life in a nursing home.

Anne Digby is Research Professor in History at Oxford Brookes University. She has published widely on the history of welfare in Britain, and on the social history of medicine in Britain, and in South Africa. Her latest book, Diversity and Division in Medicine: Healthcare in South Africa since the 1800s will be published in the Spring of 2006. Currently she is researching the history of Groote Schuur Hospital in Cape Town with colleagues from the University of Cape Town.

Elisabeth Hsu is University Lecturer at the Institute of Social and Cultural Anthropology, convenor of the M Sc and M Phil courses in Medical Anthropology, and fellow of Green College at the University of Oxford. Her main publications are: The Transmission of Chinese Medicine (1999), an ethnography of ways of learning qigong and Chinese medicine in three different social settings of Kunming City in the People's Republic of China; Innovation in Chinese Medicine (2001), an edited volume of twelve articles which testify to changing paradigms historically in Chinese medicine; and The Telling Touch (forthcoming), a translation and anthropologically framed commentary on medical case histories, body concepts and nosological entities in the biography of an ancient Chinese doctor of the second century BCE, all published with CUP.

Jenny Littlewood is formerly Research Fellow, University of London, and Reader in Primary Health Care at the South Bank University, London. She has been involved in health research from a psycho-anthropological perspective, and has been concerned with the cultural issues involved in health assessments, access and treatments, and foetal death before the medico-legal definition of life. Her publications include 'Risky shifts or shifting risk: African and African-Caribbean women's narratives on delay in seeking help for breast cancer' (with E. Elias) Risk, Decision and Policy (2000) 5: 215–224, and 'From an invisibility of miscarriage to an attribution of life' Anthropology and Medicine (1999) 6,2: 217–230.

Kent Maynard is Professor of Sociology/Anthropology as well as Director of the Honors Program at Denison University, Ohio, USA. Among other research interests, he has published widely on social identity, cultural poetics, and the nature of medicine and well-being in Cameroon. His most recent book, Making Kedjom Medicine: A History of Public Health and Well-Being in Cameroon was published with Praeger in 2004. At present, he is working on a book about agency, culture and poetics, and is conducting research on the dis/placement of medicine in West African societies.

Jan Ovesen teaches anthropology at Uppsala University. After earlier fieldwork in Afghanistan and Burkina Faso, he shifted to Southeast Asia in the mid-1990s, working in Laos and Cambodia. His main research interests are in political and medical anthropology, and ethnicity. Publications include When Every Household is an Island; Social Organization and Power Structures in Rural Cambodia (co-author, Uppsala 1996); 'Indigenous Peoples and Development in Laos – Ideologies and Ironies', in Moussons (2003); 'Foreigners and Honorary Khmers. Ethnic Minorities in Cambodia' (with I-B. Trankell), in Civilizing the Margins. Southeast Asian Government Policies for the Development of Minorities, ed. C. Duncan (Cornell University Press 2004); 'Political Violence in Cambodia and the Khmer Rouge "Genocide"', in No Peace, No War; An Anthropology of Contemporary Armed Conflicts, ed. P. Richards (James Currey 2005).

Ing-Britt Trankell teaches anthropology at Uppsala University. She has done fieldwork in northern Thailand and, since the 1990s, in Laos and Cambodia. Publications include Cooking, Care and Domestication; A Culinary Ethnography of the Tai Yong, Northern Thailand (Uppsala 1995); Facets of Power and Its Limitations; Political Culture in Southeast Asia (co-editor, Uppsala 1998); 'Royal Relics: Ritual and Social Memory in Luang Prabang', in Lao Culture and Society, ed. G. Evans (Silkworm Books 1999); 'Songs of Our Spirits: Possession and Historical Imagination among the Cham of Cambodia' in Asian Ethnicity (2003); 'French Colonial Medicine in Cambodia: Reflections of Governmentality' (with J. Ovesen), in Anthropology and Medicine (2004). She has recently completed a four-year study, with J. Ovesen, on the Indigenization of Modern Medicine in Cambodia. Focusing on the colonial, Khmer Rouge, and contemporary eras, the study is due to be published in 2006.

INDEX